PERRI KLASS is both a pediatrician and a prolific
author of fiction and nonfiction. She has published
stories and articles in *The New York Times Magazine*,
Vogue, *Mademoiselle*, *The Antioch Review*, and many
other national magazines. She has written three works
of fiction, *Other Women's Children*, *Recombinations*,
and *I Am Having an Adventure*, as well as a nonfiction
account of her work as a pediatrician, *Baby Doctor*.

A Not Entirely Benign Procedure

FOUR YEARS AS A MEDICAL STUDENT

PERRI KLASS

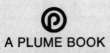

A PLUME BOOK

PLUME
Published by the Penguin Group
Penguin Books USA Inc., 375 Hudson Street, New York, New York 10014, U.S.A.
Penguin Books Ltd, 27 Wrights Lane, London W8 5TZ, England
Penguin Books Australia Ltd, Ringwood, Victoria, Australia
Penguin Books Canada Ltd, 10 Alcorn Avenue, Toronto, Ontario, Canada M4V 3B2
Penguin Books (N.Z.) Ltd, 182–190 Wairau Road, Auckland 10, New Zealand

Penguin Books Ltd, Registered Offices: Harmondsworth, Middlesex, England

Published by Plume, an imprint of Dutton Signet,
a division of Penguin Books USA Inc.
This is an authorized reprint of a hardcover edition
published by The Putnam Berkley Group Inc.

First Plume Printing, July, 1994
10 9 8 7 6 5 4 3 2 1

The author gratefully acknowledges permission from the following sources to
reprint material in their control:
Viking Penguin, Inc., for lines from *The Portable Dorothy Parker*.
Copyright © 1928, renewed 1956 by Dorothy Parker.
Tom Lehrer for lines from "The Masochism Tango." Copyright © 1958.

Ⓟ REGISTERED TRADEMARK—MARCA REGISTRADA

LIBRARY OF CONGRESS CATALOGING-IN-PUBLICATION DATA
Klass, Perri, 1958–
    A not entirely benign procedure : four years as a medical student
 / Perri Klass.
        p.   cm.
    Originally published in 1987 by Putnam, New York.
    ISBN 0-452-27258-0 (pbk.)
    1. Klass, Perri, 1958–   . 2. Medical students—Massachusetts—
Biography.   3. Harvard Medical School.   I. Title.
R154.K356A3   1994
610′.71′174461—dc20
    [B]   93–50781
                                                                    CIP
Printed in the United States of America

This book is dedicated with love
to my father, Morton Klass,
a gentleman and a scholar
if ever there was one.

Acknowledgments

In order to write this book I had to go to medical school. That was not quite how I looked at it, of course (and not quite how I said it in my medical school application essays), but there it is. In fact, in order to write this book I had to have a baby in the middle of medical school, so you can see that a great deal of labor of various kinds went into this production.

It was Susan Schneider at *Mademoiselle* magazine who first suggested that I write about medical school; earlier she had bought the first short story I ever published. At *The New York Times,* Nancy Newhouse offered me the chance to write the "Hers" column, gambling that I would manage to write coherently in the midst of the insane schedule about which I was writing. Gil Rogin at *Discover* magazine has provided me with a truly congenial home and encouraged my admittedly warped sense of humor. Also at *Discover,* Marilyn Minden has offered me careful and intelligent editing, patiently working with me over the phone in odd moments snatched out of my hospital day. Faith Sale at G. P. Putnam's Sons has been a friend and a pleasure to work with, offering me guidance, comfort, and encouragement at every turn. My agent, Maxine Groffsky, is really directly responsible for this book's existence; she thought I could write columns, and she thought people might want to read them. I am extremely grateful to her for everything—and also for taking it all in the right spirit. Finally, I am grateful to William Abrahams, who has given me great encouragement and invaluable advice.

But I did have to go to medical school. There have been

several people who by encouragement or example helped me through. In my very first year, as I looked around in confusion, wondering where I was and what I was doing there, Pearl O'Rourke offered me, every week, a chance to see why a doctor's life might be both rewarding and fascinating. Also, it was good to know there was someone out there with a sense of humor even more warped than my own. Orah Platt, who was my academic advisor, and also my friend and my support during the dark days of internship application, is another wonderful pediatrician. I know that I went into pediatrics partly because of these teachers of mine; I also know that in the way they thought and spoke and acted, they countermanded everything disturbing or disillusioning about medical school.

I owe a very special gratitude to the various classmates, residents, and attendants who wittingly or unwittingly provided me with all my best material. I owe a different kind of gratitude to Mitch Katz. Not that he didn't give me material—most of the best jokes in this book are his—but he also helped me through medical school. Although our joint project, a guide to restaurants near the Harvard teaching hospitals that are accessible for lunch (especially if you take a two-and-a-half-hour break), has yet to be published, I would certainly never have graduated without those lunches. There were many days when I learned as much medicine from our intense and scholarly lunchtime discussions as I did from the day's lectures.

My parents, Morton and Sheila Klass, have done a tremendous amount for me. First, I freely admit: they never particularly wanted me to go to medical school. They did, however, allow themselves to be exploited, as I applied to medical school and then bopped off to Italy for a year, leaving them to cope with admissions committees and form letters and transcript requests. And they got in! I mean, they got me in. And they have paid large sums of exorbitant tuition, for a daughter who ought to have been old enough to support herself. And they have listened to me complain, accepted grouchy collect calls from the hospital in the middle of the night. And they have nodded and looked impressed whenever I showed off newly acquired medical knowledge. In short, they have encouraged me, supported me, humored me, comforted me, and put up with me. No one could possibly have better parents.

Larry Wolff, five years ago, typed my medical school application essay as I stormed around the room in a neurotic frenzy. He lived with me through medical school, which was not all fun and games. I whined, I worried, I became desperately anxious about exams when it was too late to study and miserably insecure about the hospital during my few hours outside it. No one should have to live with a medical student. But Larry did it, and with grace, kindness, and good nature. Without Larry, there would have been little pleasure, little happiness, and probably no writing. He got me through medical school, with no small effort. He has also put endless time and energy into my writing, and this book owes much to him, always the first and sharpest reader of anything I write.

Our son, Benjamin Orlando Klass, was born halfway through my medical school training. He has brought, from the beginning, nothing but delight. Medical school would have been no fun at all without Benjamin.

Contents

Introduction

I did not originally intend to go to medical school, and when I started medical school, I certainly did not intend to write about it. I had majored in biology in college, thinking at first about becoming a doctor, but moved off in the direction of biological research. I began to picture myself going into the jungle to study animals, and so I took the first step toward the jungle and went off to graduate school in zoology. The animals I chose to study were parasitic organisms, and I was interested in questions of ecology and evolution as applied to parasites; I wondered how a life cycle could evolve that required two, or even three, different hosts, all synchronized into the development of the parasite. But hanging around parasitology you meet a lot of doctors and biomedical researchers, and after a couple of years I decided that I was interested in the human hosts as well as the parasites, so I applied to medical school. I make it all sound casual and a little light-hearted; in fact I had to put a great deal of effort into areas in which I am not talented—notably learning enough chemistry and physics to do decently on the eight-hour multiple-choice test required of all medical school applicants. I had come close to flunking these courses in college and needed to convince medical schools that I had since learned the material. I filled in applications, and when the time came I bought a suit and flew around the country for interviews. I smiled and looked enthusiastic and got asked all sorts of exciting questions, including why had I almost failed chemistry and physics in college (I rehearsed a good many answers to that one, finally went with a disarmingly sincere statement about being out of my depth back in those first years of college, and simply not knowing how to study properly—it wasn't exactly true, but it was disarmingly sincere). I toured any number of medical schools, asking the questions applicants all ask on these tours, most notably, "How many students to a cadaver?" At some schools it's four, at others it's five or six. Is this a basis on which to choose your medical school? No, but it's one of the few questions for which you can get a firm objective answer. I no longer remember which schools have how many students to a cadaver.

I have been writing for most of my life; I come from a family in which most people write, and publish (though no one makes a living at it), and I had been writing fiction all through high school, college, and graduate school. It never occurred to me that I wouldn't go on writing fiction in medical school, and it never occurred to me that I might start writing nonfiction. The summer before I started medical school, I achieved my first publication: a story of mine was printed in *Mademoiselle* magazine. Although I was of course pleased to get into medical school, I have to say that the acceptance from *Mademoiselle* was easily ten times as exciting. I mean, it's hard to get into medical school, but thousands of people do it every year.

I had gone to college at Harvard, then moved out to Berkeley for graduate school. The year I was applying to medical school, I took some time off from school of any kind and went to Italy with my friend Larry Wolff. He researched his doctoral dissertation in the Vatican archives while I worked in a lab and did some writing.

In September of 1982, we moved back to Cambridge, Massachusetts, and settled in.

Medical school was sort of a great unknown for me. No one in my family had ever gone, and for the last few years I had been hanging out with graduate students. I didn't know what to expect, and I had only limited confidence that the process was going to be successful, that I was going to come out the other end a real doctor. Most of what I knew about medicine was what I had seen on television; as a child, I had been a great devotee of *Marcus Welby, M.D.,* and *Medical Center.* But I started medical school without any very clear idea of what my training would be like, of what would come after medical school, of what choices I might have in front of me.

Toward the end of my first year of medical school, an editor at *Mademoiselle* suggested that I write an article for the magazine about being a woman in the first year of medical school. I had never written anything like this before, and I more or less blundered my way through it. The article was published, and later I was offered other opportunities to write about my training. I had entered a world which was as mysterious to most people as it had been for me, and it seemed that there were readers interested in hearing the details. I wrote a weekly column in *The New York Times* for nine weeks, then later began doing regular columns for two other magazines, *Discover,* aimed at a general readership interested in science, and *Massachusetts Medicine,* which goes to doctors and medical students. I have also done articles for a variety of other publications.

Meanwhile, I went through medical school. I also had a baby; I got pregnant toward the end of my first year and had the baby in the middle of the second year, and I ended up writing about that too.

The experience of writing about medical school while

going through it has changed my medical education tremendously. I have found that in order to write about my training so that people outside the medical profession can understand what I am talking about I have had to preserve a certain level of naiveté for myself. I have to hear and see things not only as a doctor, who would take most hospital sights, most medical locutions, completely for granted, but also as a nondoctor. Instead of trying to forget, as quickly as possible, what it felt like to be in the operating room for the first time (Who are all these people? What are they doing? What are all these machines? What are those tubes for? Where am I supposed to stand? What am I supposed to do? This is completely disgusting; what if I faint?), I had to try to preserve all those disorienting sensations and impressions.

The general pressure in medical school is to push yourself ahead into professionalism, to start feeling at home in the hospital, in the operating room, to make medical jargon your native tongue—it's all part of becoming efficient, knowledgeable, competent. You want to leave behind that green, terrified medical student who stood awkwardly on the edge of the action, terrified of revealing limitless ignorance, terrified of killing a patient. You want to identify with the people ahead of you, the ones who know what they're doing. And instead, I have found it necessary to retain some of that greenness, so I could explain the hospital to people for whom it was not familiar turf.

Of course, it becomes a little artificial after a while, and there are sensations I can no longer remember. The hospital no longer feels alien or threatening to me, the medical jargon is familiar in my ears. Once you have come to understand a language, it is probably impossible to recapture exactly what it felt like to hear it as gibberish.

There are things I find funny which are funny only

to doctors or medical students. I can laugh at a fellow student doing an imitation of an inept medical student trying and trying to draw blood from a patient; I laugh in recognition, in identification with the student, but nondoctors cringe in horror, identifying with the poor abused patient. And so I have to acknowledge that despite a very deliberate attempt to remember the perceptions of someone without medical training, I have in fact become someone with medical training, and with the attendant perceptions.

The essays in this book were written during the four years I spent in medical school. The essay about the first year was in fact written at the end of my first year. The essay on beginning clinical training, drawing blood from a patient for the first time, was written during my first months in the hospital. I have not altered these pieces to make them more uniform, because it seems to me that if my voice has changed through medical school, then that change should be part of the education process I have been writing about.

Medical school divides into two parts. For the first two years, I was mostly in the classroom, listening to lectures, carrying out various kinds of lab exercises (looking at slides under a microscope, dissecting a cadaver). Then the second two years I was "on the wards," in the hospitals. I spent a month or two in each of a number of specialties, a month in radiology, two months in surgery, a month in psychiatry, and so on. And sometime during this clinical training, I decided what branch of medicine I wanted to enter—pediatrics.

This outline of my medical education also provides a general outline for this book. The first section concerns the classroom training, the pre-clinical years. Then comes a section of essays about the actual hands-on learning of clinical medicine, my experiences on the wards. The third section is made up of essays about specific medical issues, many of them controversial, that I was exposed to as a medical student. And in the last section I have tried to sum up my experiences: the science, the clinical training, the various ethical and medical dilemmas. I wanted to attempt some sort of stocktaking, some assessment of the training I have received and will continue to receive.

These essays add up to a record of medical school for me; they describe not only my experiences but also the various preoccupations that buzzed in my head as I ran around the hospital in my white coat, stethoscope flapping, trying to take care of "my" patients, make good impressions on the right people, learn a little medicine, and get a little sleep. I have not been an exemplary medical student, and I do not feel, looking back, that I have necessarily taken advantage of all the opportunities to learn that came my way. On the other hand, I didn't kill anyone, and I didn't crack up, and I didn't lose my sense of humor (though I am afraid it's gotten a little bit twisted), so my worst fears didn't come true either.

Over the past couple of years, as I have published the various pieces collected here, I have received a good deal of mail. Much of it has been interesting, some has been hostile. I have been accused a number of times, by doctors and medical students, of presenting the medical profession in a bad light. These were letters from sane people who happened to disagree with me.

Recently, I have been the target of a very different kind of letterwriting. Someone has written to the editors of all the magazines I contribute to, accusing me of having plagiarized my articles. These letters purported to be from a variety of different people; the writer claimed in different letters to be a relative of one of my classmates, a nurse, an interested bystander, and, finally, actually to have attended medical school with me. "Evidence" to back up the accusation of plagiarism (or, as this creature prefers to call it, plagiarization) was provided in the form of supposed "originals," the articles from which I had copied—but these originals were photocopies of unidentified articles from unidentified magazines; the author of the anonymous letters claimed to have these original articles but just happened not to know where they came from.

In other words, someone had gone to the trouble of copying bits out of my articles and having them typeset so they looked as though they had been printed in a different form. In one case, most of an article of mine had been rewritten into a piece supposedly authored by a student nurse in England during the Second World War. Many little changes had been made to give verisimilitude to this claim—though many words and phrases remained more suited to an American medical student in the 1980s. Again there was no reference, no way to trace the purported "source," but the fabrication had plainly taken a good deal of trouble and effort on the part of someone who was not stupid, but also not precisely sane.

If I had any doubts about the mental stability (not to mention good taste) of my persecutor, they were resolved when I was sent, at the same time those letters were received, a gift-wrapped ribbon-tied box of human excrement.

Plagiarism is of course the easiest thing in the world to prove—if you can produce the original piece of writing. When anonymous letters and "originals" without references failed to discredit me, the letters were sent to a wider range of people—to nurses at the hospital where I work, to newspapers and magazines in the Boston area. The accusations increased in number and scope: Perri Klass boasts about her plagiarizations. She eagerly demonstrates to all comers just how she cheated on her physiology exam. Everyone who went to medical school with her knew that other people's experiments weren't safe if she was around. And finally, inevitably, when nothing else seemed to provoke the desired response: she's medically incompetent, a danger to her patients.

This has been, as you might imagine, a very unpleasant experience. It isn't comfortable to know that somebody out there hates you that much. You can't help feeling that if enough mud is slung, some of it may stick. One suggestion made repeatedly by the people investigating this campaign was that the creature writing the letters was someone inside the medical profession. Maybe someone who really had gone to medical school with me, maybe someone who hadn't made it—there was evidence that whoever it was knew something about hospitals, about my medical school class. And in my darker moments, I sometimes wonder whether this campaign, on which some pathetic and probably demented person is lavishing so much time and attention, has its roots in someone's sense that I have betrayed my profession. There are things you aren't supposed to say to nondoctors, things they aren't supposed to know.

The pieces in this book come so very directly out of my own experience that the whole issue of plagiarism feels somehow out of place. When I showed friends one fabricated "original," a paragraph I was accused of having copied, supposedly published years before my classmates and I started medical school, we were all amazed to see that what it described was a clinic we all remembered well from our first year of medical school. It was hard not to wonder whether the motive behind the fabrication was not only to do me damage but also to deny my right to describe my own experiences—perhaps because they had also been my accuser's experiences, and I had violated them, criticized them, opened them up to nondoctors.

Of course, this may not be true. I may never know what motivated this person—what does it take to make even a disturbed person neatly gift-wrap a box of excrement? I am only following the ideas suggested by the detectives—and some suspicions of my own.

The one bright spot in this tense and unhappy episode has been that I have been able to turn to one of my favorite books. *Gaudy Night* by Dorothy L. Sayers is mentioned later on in one of the essays as a book which I often use for emotional support of one kind or another. The heroine of this novel is the target of many anonymous letters, which she judges and deals with briskly. Early in the book, she finds an unpleasant drawing:

"It was neither sane nor healthy; it was, in fact, a nasty, dirty and lunatic scribble.

"Harriet stared at it for a little time in disgust, while a number of questions formed themselves in her mind. Then she took it upstairs with her into the nearest lavatory, dropped it in and pulled the plug on it. That was the proper fate for such things, and there was an end of it; but for all that, she wished she had not seen it."

THE PRE-CLINICAL YEARS

A liberal education had of course left him free to read
the indecent passages in the school classics, but beyond
a general sense of secrecy and obscenity in connection
with his internal structure, had left his imagination
quite unbiassed, so that for anything he knew his
brains lay in small bags at his temples, and he had no
more thought of representing to himself how his blood
circulated than how paper served instead of gold.

GEORGE ELIOT, *Middlemarch*

THE FIRST TWO YEARS of medical school are the pre-clinical years, the years before you get out into the hospitals. During the first year, we focused on basic biology, anatomy, physiology, cell biology—the science of the normal body. We were supposed to come out with an understanding of how the body is put together and how it functions. The first year of medical school is also often seen as one of those traditional "proving grounds," like the first year of law school, like basic training—it is when you supposedly learn the standards of your new society, measure yourself against expectations which will exceed anything you have encountered before. On the other hand, at my medical school (among others) there are no letter grades, so the first year of medical school is a time when people who have been killing themselves to do well in their premed courses are supposed to relax and learn the material for its own sake. It's pass/fail, and, as the class ahead of us told us, remember the equation: $P = MD$. Of course, it is possible to fail (in which case you have to retake the exam and if necessary the course). And in fact, many courses are graded pass/fail/excellent, so if you are so inclined you can focus on those "excellents" and treat medical school with the same kind of competitiveness that has made the premed curriculum legendary.

In the second year of medical school, the emphasis

was on disease, pathophysiology. The courses dealt with one organ system after another, the heart, the gastrointestinal system, the reproductive system, and so on. And for each system, we learned every possible malfunction, the congenital defects, the infections, the tumors. This two-year program left me with what is referred to as my basic fund of knowledge, my basic science and my pathophysiology. It was two years of relatively rigorous classroom and laboratory learning, with occasional exposure to real patients, usually a patient speaking to a large group of medical students. More often, we studied case problems, descriptions of patients, which stopped after every few pieces of information to ask, what would you do now? what tests would you order? what questions would you ask? how would you treat?

This section consists of two long articles, one about each of those two long years of study. The first is a general piece about my experiences during my first year, my impressions of this introduction to a new world. The article about my second year focuses on a somewhat atypical aspect of that year—I had a baby in the middle of it. I found that my pregnancy, which turned me into a "patient," changed the way I viewed the teaching and learning of pathophysiology.

At the end of my second year, I took a course called "Introduction to Clinical Medicine," in which I learned, step by step, how to perform a physical examination and how to take a medical history from a patient. In order to learn the physical examination, my classmates and I practiced on each other, trying to learn how to use our brand-new stethoscopes and ophthalmoscopes. We then graduated to interviewing and examining hospital patients, under more or less careful supervision. And then we were judged ready to enter the next stage of our training: the clinical years.

I found the first two years of medical school a difficult but not horrible experience. It was frequently (especially during the first year) hard to remember exactly why I was doing this, what the connection was to medicine. Academically, the courses were not impossibly demanding. It was perfectly possible to have a baby. However, the experience of being socialized into a medical school class was at times disturbing, as was the strong sense that values were being taught, though not explicitly, along with the basic science and pathophysiology.

The pre-clinical years were an initiation. Not into the hospital; that came later. But by the time I got to the hospital, I was no longer a complete outsider, and the difference was not only that I knew some pathophysiology. The initiation went deeper than that, and in these articles, each written right after the period it describes, I tried to explain what was happening to me. I couldn't write either of those pieces now, even a couple of years later, because I have totally lost track of what it felt like to be what I suppose I have to call pre-clinical.

The Living-in-Sin Potluck and Other Tales of the First Year of Medical School

The beginning of my first year at Harvard Medical School. Orientation, speeches, barbecues. Slowly I am meeting my classmates, about a hundred forty of them. They seem like a pleasant group, most of them just out of college, excited about starting something new. I am terrified of them. I am terrified of my classes. I am terrified that in the three years since I graduated from college I have simply lost the ability to keep up with regular homework assignments and quizzes, midterms and labs. I have a guilty secret as well: in college, I was a very slipshod sort of student. My "study habits," such as they were, were the last-minute-scramble, stay-up-all-night-and-panic kind. They got me through college, though not without pain, but I am sure they will never work in medical school. All of these fresh-faced young people around me must be perfect studiers, demons for organization. In my terror, I begin to make resolutions. I make little charts of how I will arrange my studying time: every night I will review the material from that day's lectures and then go over the material for the next day. At the end of every week I will do a major review of the whole week's work. I breathe a sigh of pleasure and relief as I picture the neat pages of notes I will make, the textbooks carefully underlined and annotated. I will not fall behind. I will not cut classes. I will like myself; I will feel that glow of self-satisfaction that I am sure "good students" feel.

It takes only a week or two for things to get back to normal. I stop going to the 8:30 lectures because the minute they turn off the lights to show slides I fall fast asleep. Clearly I am better off at home in bed. Falling behind becomes an irrelevant concept; I can't even imagine what it would mean to be caught up. And, just as in college, I continue to do fine, studying ferociously at the last minute for exams, cutting classes, and doing the reading on my own. But unfortunately, just as in college, I feel perpetually dissatisfied with myself; somewhere out there, I am sure, are my class-mates, doing all of this the *right* way.

Physiology, histology, biochemistry, neurobiology. The first semester is under way. I am beginning to know some of my classmates, I know the locker com-bination to get out my microscope, I am even learning where the women's bathrooms are (second floor, Build-ing E, but third floor, Building A . . .). I must say, I feel a little bit like I am back in high school. There are no decisions to make; I simply march through the day in step with the other people in my class; we go from lecture to lab to lunch to lecture together. This can be monotonous, but I also find it reassuring; I will sit here passively and they will turn me into a doctor. This metamorphosis is a miracle which will be worked upon my acquiescent, receptive body and mind.

And then I have to make a decision, my whole class has to make a decision, and it turns into a collective trauma. The trauma of "dog lab." Dog lab is a lab we are all supposed to do in connection with what we have been learning in physiology about the cardiovas-cular system. Essentially, dog lab means that a group of four medical students will spend six hours perform-ing various experiments on the heart and circulatory system of an anesthetized dog. At the end of the afternoon, the dog is dead, and the medical students, in theory, have a much fuller appreciation of the functioning of the heart.

And so I finally do have a decision to make: am I going to do this lab? I am not a vegetarian, I am not a passionate dog-lover, I am not opposed to animal experimentation on principle. I envy my classmates who are any or all of these things; their decisions must be so straightforward.

"The idea of doing the lab bothers me, that's all." That's what I end up saying to my classmates, to my parents, to friends who don't go to medical school. These friends are invariably horrified by the very idea of the lab ("You dissect it while it's still *alive*?"), and yet somehow I feel their horror is not the same as mine. They make me wonder: have I crossed some dividing line already, that I can even consider doing this thing?

I think it is very ugly that this lab should come along so early in my medical education. Why should I be beginning my training with the prolonged killing of an animal? I worry so much, as it is, about the unpleasant and painful things I will see later on in my training and in my career. I am scared that in order to handle them, I will have to become "toughened" in ways I won't like. Isn't there something wrong with starting off by causing pain without any intention to cure?

And then I worry that this is all hysterical nonsense, that I am passing up an incredible learning experience because of absurd scruples about killing a completely anesthetized dog which comes from the pound and would be killed anyway. I wake up in the middle of the night dreaming about dogs or surgery; I keep waiting for a dream in which dogs are operating on me. I find myself talking about the subject obsessively; I have to be told by some non–medical student friends that they find it an inappropriate topic for dinner-table conversation. I am becoming a bore, I think.

Meanwhile, at the medical school, the students who are definitely planning to do the lab are beginning to say to the people who think they won't, "How are you ever going to be a doctor if you're too sensitive to do dog lab? How are you going to take it when you're in the hospitals?" Some of the women in my class are particularly vulnerable to this kind of reasoning; they worry that they aren't tough enough, that they cannot afford to pass up any opportunity to prove, to themselves and to everyone else, that they have what it takes. In some ways, it is this kind of thing that finally decides me not to do the lab. It's a confirmation of all my worst suspicions—this lab is intended to toughen me, to divide me from ordinary normal people.

So I make my decision, and I do shut up about it. But it keeps on waking me up at night. Am I doing the right thing, after all? I find myself sitting on a friend's floor at a potluck brunch, listening to a man in my class lecturing me about what a valuable learning experience the lab would be for me. He is pompous and very boring (have I been sounding like *that*?). I tell him I've made up my mind to learn the material from other sources. And he says to me, "You really think you know more about it than Harvard Medical School? You think you know more about medical education than they do?"

Well, there are several responses to this, beyond the obvious one, "What a turkey this guy is!" I guess I have come to the conclusion that yes, I do know more about how *I* learn than Harvard Medical School does. I am amazed that after the relatively indifferent teaching we have been receiving for the past month or so, this man is speaking of the school in terms of holy awe. I am amazed that after a month he identifies himself so absolutely with the institution. And I am more than a little amazed that I am still so absorbed in this issue that I am willing to sit here discussing it with this guy, who is, after all, a turkey.

There is a married students' association at the medical school, but they are not eager to have students who are only engaged (much less just living together) come to their functions. So one day a medical student gets up in front of the class and announces the first Living-in-Sin Potluck.

(In medical school, the potlucks are nonstop. Off-campus potluck, women's potluck, housewarming potluck—no one should go to medical school without a couple of really reliable recipes.) And so "those of us who are sharing these special years with someone to whom we are less formally bound," as the organizer says, honor our partners and each other one evening in the spring. And the medical students complain about medical school, and the partners complain about living with medical students, and a good time is had by all.

I am not easy to live with this year. I am always worrying about one test or another, I am always talking about things that don't really mean much to non-medical students ("I mean, can you believe it? Every single problem on that problem set used those respiratory equations we haven't even learned yet!"), and, most of all I am very busy. And I am more than a little self-righteous about my busyness. Of course I can't do the shopping, I'm a medical sudent. Of course I can't wash the dishes, I have studying to do. All this is quite unpleasant for the man I live with, who objects, legitimately, to living in a perpetual state of crisis. It's one thing for him to take tender loving care of me when I'm actually in the middle of exam period, but as an everyday state of affairs, it's a little wearing. I do begin to understand the assumption on which many male doctors have always operated: one medical career requires two lives. A doctor needs a full-time wife. I can feel myself developing the attitude that my work is so much more important than what anyone else is doing that naturally those who live with me should be downright honored to help me in my great task—"What great task are we talking about here?" asks the man I live with. "Passing the biochemistry midterm?" Over the course of the year, I slowly begin to do a little more toward keeping our apartment in shape, toward shopping and cooking and laundry. I try to edit my conversation. What will be interesting for a "normal person" to hear about? Have I been talking about medical school for the last half hour?

And sometimes it occurs to me that I am in fact tremendously lucky to be living with someone who doesn't go to medical school. If it weren't for him, would I even remember that there is a world out there full of people who don't care about the equations on my respiratory physiology problem set?

"The lack of female role models" is a phrase I have heard so often that I am tired of it, but it is a very real lack. I am very lucky to have a clinical tutor, a doctor who meets once a week with me and three other students and takes us around the hospital, who does provide me with a strongly positive role model. Her manner is devoid of the kind of stiffness and cold formality that it seems many doctors put on with the white coat (or are they like that all the time?). She works in a pediatric intensive care ward, so her patients are children who are terribly sick, children who have been in serious accidents, children born with severe birth defects. I watch her hands as she touches these children. Will I ever possess that kind of competence, that kind of sure ability to help and comfort? How can I ever learn it? Watching her, I think that being a doctor, a good doctor, would be the most wonderful thing I could possibly do with my life.

And yet spending time in the pediatric intensive care ward is the most disturbing thing I do all year. There is too much drama, too much tragedy. I look at the very small children with tubes going into them, with machines hooked up to them, and I want to protest that it just isn't *fair*. I am very shaken by the grisly evidence of how thin the barrier is between normal life and disaster. These parents had a normal, happy, healthy daughter until yesterday when she was crossing the street and was hit by a car. Will she ever come out of the coma? This family had an active two-year-old son until two days ago. Now they are waiting to see how much brain function he can hope to recover. The stories sound like soap opera, of course. Maybe what gets to me is the sense of how quickly life can become soap opera.

I watch my tutor and her colleagues. Obviously they have developed some self-protective mechanisms. Children die in this ward, and the doctors and nurses can't collapse every time it happens. And yet they are not quite as protected as I might have expected. They are very depressed sometimes when things go badly. And on the other hand there is the day my tutor ushers us into a room to see a girl the doctors had practically given up for dead, but who has rallied and is now sitting up in bed cheerfully talking to her mother. When my tutor introduces us to this girl and then says to us with an enormous grin, *"This* is the beauty of pediatrics!" it is clear that she does not take these triumphs for granted any more than she does the failures.

I have nightmares about tubes, machines, dying children. I go home from the hospital every week wondering whether I'll ever be able to handle this. And yet this is also the time every week when I am most confident that I have chosen the right profession.

Gross anatomy. All year, whenever I tell people I go to medical school, they ask me about cutting up a cadaver. In fact, at Harvard we don't do that until the second semester. We have already, as a class, undergone another collective trauma: we have chosen dissection partners for anatomy. We were all obsessed with the decision, evidence once more of how the little issues of medical school have come to dominate our lives. We are given so few decisions that each one takes on enormous weight. We discussed it endlessly. Should you dissect with your best friend? Should you dissect with someone you might be romantically interested in? Should you dissect with someone who is a more conscientious or a less conscientious student than you are? Tearful phone calls. Confrontations in the hallways. Diplomacy, deals, betrayals.

Finally it is the first day and we stand in the anatomy lab in white coats and plastic aprons and plastic gloves. Each group of four students stands around a metal table, and on each metal table is a cadaver covered with a cloth. The cloths, incongruously, are made of denim. We are all very much aware that in a few minutes they will tell us to take off the cloths. The room is cold and quiet; we are all scared, I think. For the very first time in medical school, I have a sense that I am being initiated into a priesthood. This is something that "normal people" never do. There is a body on this table which was once alive and is now dead, and I am going to take it apart, and somehow I am going to come away understanding much more about both life and death. We take off the cloths.

And so we do the first dissection, opening up the chest of our cadaver. The skin, after long soaking in formaldehyde, is quite leathery; it doesn't look or feel like skin, which makes it easier to cut. Our cadaver is female, and when the time comes to cut away the breast, I feel a certain tremor in my own chest. In fact, none of the four of us, three women and one man, is eager to do that, and we find ourselves delaying until one of the teachers comes around and does it for us.

The semester moves on. I do like anatomy. I find myself watching the muscles move under my own skin when I flex my arm, thinking about how they attach to bones, how they are nourished by blood vessels, how the nerves weave in and out. In fact, when the exam comes, we are all sitting there flexing and extending our limbs, trying to remember which muscle fits in where. One man with a very well developed upper body comes to the exam in a tight sleeveless teeshirt, and all the students sitting near him keep sneaking surreptitious looks at his biceps, his triceps, his pecs.

One unpleasant thing about taking anatomy is the smell. We all stink. The formaldehyde penetrates my hair and clothes, right through the plastic apron and the white coat and the two pairs of gloves and the layer of skin cream. Sometimes at night, after I have washed my hair, I am sure that I catch a persistent whiff of formaldehyde, and I want to apologize; it can't be particularly delightful to share a bed with someone who smells faintly of cadavers.

I am lucky though; gross anatomy doesn't disturb me. There are people who dream about cadavers and people who dread each day's dissecting. I know that because I don't mind it I am giving myself credit for having passed another "toughness test" and I know just how ridiculous that is; it's no virtue of mine if this doesn't happen to bother me. And yet when I sympathize with friends who hate it, I am always conscious of a faint patronizing quality in my voice. I do find, by the way, that I can't eat meat on the days we dissect; it just looks too familiar. So it's always possible to find a test I'll fail.

Medical students taking anatomy. There are all kinds of stories about the jokes, the crudity, the coarse humor. Some of it is not deliberate; the man I live with has to point out to me a number of times that there are certain details he would rather not hear ("So we were cleaning the fat away from the stomach muscles and all of a sudden . . ."). By and large, the humor in the dissecting room itself is more at the expense of the medical students than at the expense of the cadaver. In spite of everything, I continue to feel that we are treating our cadaver with some respect and even perhaps with some awe. It is hard for me to think of it (her?) as a living person, but when I do, I think of her with gratitude: she was genuinely generous with herself, and because of that generosity, I am learning things I would never have been able to learn in any other way.

But of course there is a certain amount of dissecting-room humor. For example, there is the day we come in to do the dissection of the male reproductive system and notice that all the men in the class are looking pretty green. The women students get to do a lot of dissecting that particular day; the men are not eager to do any cutting. And, I have to admit it, we do make jokes. My group of four "cadaver-mates" is sent to dissect one of the testicles of a different cadaver, since ours is female. The four of us are all crouched over what is, after all, a very small structure, when my partner says thoughtfully, "You know, this is a good metaphor for life." We all straighten up and look at her quizzically. "Well," she says, gesturing, "in order to get anything done in life, you have to push the penis out of the way."

To be fair, I and many of the other women find the dissection of the female reproductive system somewhat more difficult emotionally. It's hard to cut up structures about which you feel very protective; it's a lot easier with structures you simply don't possess.

I have to wonder, of course: is there some clue there to the way the medical profession has always treated women?

My clinical tutor has arranged a meeting with a woman whose child is dying of cancer. She is willing to talk to some medical students about how she and her family are handling the situation. Before we go up to meet her, our tutor says, "This is an intelligent, articulate woman. Be sensitive when you talk to her. Don't spend any time on the scientific aspects of the disease; we can go over that later. What I want you to get from talking to her is some appreciation of what this kind of sickness does to a whole family." So we go upstairs and meet this woman in one of the playrooms in the pediatric oncology unit. There are two medical students, me and a man in my class.

He asks the first question. "So in this kind of cancer, what's going on with the immune system? The B cells, for example, are they being synthesized abnormally?"

Our tutor cuts in, reminds him that we can go over the technical details later on. He considers for a minute, then asks another question, equally scientific. Our tutor cuts in again. My fellow medical student is perplexed. It's perfectly clear that he can't imagine what kinds of questions she has in mind—what other kinds of interesting questions are there? He shuts up altogether, and my tutor, the mother, and I talk for a little while about what is happening to this two-year-old girl, and to her parents. The mother is indeed an articulate and intelligent woman, and she has a great deal she wants to say. She is eager to explain the kinds of comfort she is able to give her daughter in the hospital. She is willing to talk about how she and her husband keep going in the face of this tragedy. She is very impressive and very moving.

The other medical student gets the idea. He thinks of a question. "Do you feel really guilty about this?" he asks. "I mean, do you worry a lot about whether something you did might have caused your daughter's cancer?"

Early in the year, I ask a woman how she decided to come to Harvard Medical School (it's the sort of boring question you sometimes find yourself asking at a potluck). She is the most outrageous dresser in our class; that day she is wearing a purple minidress and fishnet stockings. "Oh," she says, "I came here because I always wanted to dye my hair pink. I figure that if I come from Harvard Medical School, I can have pink hair and people will still have to take me seriously."

This reminds me a little of why I and many other people I know came here: we want to be able to do what we want. I want to be a doctor who fits my own definition of a good doctor, and if that conflicts with other doctors' ideas, well, I want to have such impeccable credentials that they will still have to take me seriously. But the question is, by the time I finish, will I still remember any of what I originally wanted to be? When I am through with my training, will I have any way of knowing what kind of doctor I have actually become?

Later on in the year I am talking to that same woman. Teasing her, I say, "I see you still haven't dyed your hair pink."

"No," she says, with a sigh. "You see how I've been co-opted?" Then she grins at me. "I still want to, though."

A Textbook Pregnancy

I learned I was pregnant the afternoon of my anatomy exam. I had spent the morning taking first a written exam and then a practical, centered around fifteen thoroughly dissected cadavers, each ornamented with little paper tags indicating structures to be identified.

My classmates and I were not looking very good, our hair unwashed, our faces pale from too much studying and too little sleep. Two more exams and our first year of medical school would be over. We all knew exactly what we had to do next: go home and study for tomorrow's exam. I could picture my genetics notes lying on my desk, liberally highlighted with pink marker. But before I went home I had a pregnancy test done.

My period was exactly one day late, hardly worth noticing—but the month before, for the first time in my life, I had been trying to get pregnant. Four hours later I called for the test results.

"It's positive," the woman at the lab told me.

With all the confidence of a first-year medical student, I asked, "Positive, what does that mean?"

"It means you're pregnant," she told me. "Congratulations."

Somewhat later that afternoon I settled down to make final review notes for my genetics exam. *Down's syndrome,* I copied carefully onto a clean piece of paper, *most common autosomal disorder, 1 per 700 live births.* I began to feel a little queasy. Over the next twenty-four hours, I was supposed to learn the biological basis, symptoms, diagnosis, and treatment of a long list of genetic disorders. Almost every one was something that could conceivably already be wrong with the embryo growing inside me. I couldn't even think about it; I had to put my notes aside and pass the exam on what I remembered from the lectures.

Over the past months, as I have gone through my pregnancy, and also through my second year of medical school, I have become more and more aware of these two aspects of my life influencing each other, and even sometimes seeming to oppose each other. As a medical student, I was spending my time studying everything that can go wrong with the human body. As a pregnant woman, I was suddenly passionately interested in healthy physiological processes, in my own normal pregnancy and the growth of my baby. And yet pregnancy put me under the care of the medical profession—my own future profession—and I found myself rebelling as a mother and a patient against the attitudes that were being taught to me, particularly the attitude that pregnancy is a perilous, if not pathological, condition. The pregnancy and the decisions I had to make about my own health care changed my feelings about medicine and about the worldview of emergency and intervention which is communicated in medical training. My pregnancy became for me a rebellion against this worldview, a chance to do something healthy and normal with my body, something that would be a joyous event, an important event, a complex event, but not necessarily a medical event.

Medical school lasts four years, followed by internship and residency—three years for medicine, five to seven for surgery. And then maybe a two-year fellowship.

"The fellowship years can be a good time to have a baby," advised one physician. She was just finishing a fellowship in primary care. "Not internship or residency, God knows—that's when everyone's marriage breaks up since you're working eighty hours a week and you're so miserable all the time."

I am twenty-six. After college, I didn't go straight to medical school, but spent two years doing graduate work in biology and one living abroad. I'll probably have reached the fellowship stage by around thirty-three. It seemed like a long time to wait.

The more I thought about it, the more it seemed to me that there was no time in the next seven or so years when it would be as feasible to have a baby as it is now. As a medical student, I have a flexibility that I will not really have further on, a freedom to take a couple of months off or even a year if I decide I need it, and without unduly disrupting the progress of my career. Larry, who is also twenty-six, has just finished his doctoral dissertation on Polish-Vatican relations in the late eighteenth century, and is teaching at Harvard. He also has a great deal of flexibility. Both our lives frequently feel a little frantic, but we don't find ourselves looking ahead to a less complex, less frantic future.

I decided not to take a leave of absence this year. Instead, Larry and I have started on the juggling games which will no doubt be a major feature of the years ahead; I took extra courses last year so I could manage a comparatively light schedule this spring and stay with the baby two days a week while Larry worked at home for the other three. Perfect timing is of course of the essence; happily, we'd already managed to conceive the baby so it would be born between the time I took my exams in December and the time I started work at the hospital in March.

There was one other factor in my decision to have a

baby now. All through my first year of medical school, in embryology, in genetics, even in public health, lecturers kept emphasizing that the ideal time to have a baby is around the age of twenty-four. Safest for the mother. Safest for the baby. "Do you think they're trying to tell us something?" grumbled one of my classmates after a particularly pointed lecture. "Like why are we wasting these precious childbearing years in school? It almost makes you feel guilty about waiting to have children."

Ironically, I know no one else my age who is having a baby. The women in my childbirth class were all in their mid-thirties. "Having a baby is a very nineteen-eighties thing to do," said a friend who is a twenty-seven-year-old corporate lawyer in New York. "The only thing is, you and Larry are much too young." In medical school one day last month, a lecturer mentioned the problem of teenage pregnancy, and I imagined that my classmates were turning to look at me.

In theory, medical education teaches first about normal anatomy, normal physiology, and then builds upon this foundation by teaching the processes of pathology and disease. In practice, everyone—student and teacher alike—is eager to get to the material with "clinical relevance" and the whole thrust of the teaching is toward using examples of disease to illustrate normal body functions by showing what happens when such functions break down. This is the way much of medical knowledge is garnered, after all—we understand sugar metabolism partially because of studies on diabetics, who can't metabolize sugar normally. "An experiment of nature" is the phrase often used.

Although we had learned a great deal about disease, we had not, in our first year of medical school, learned much about the nitty-gritty of medical practice. As I began to wonder more about what was happening inside me and about what childbirth would be like, I tried to read my embryology textbook, but again the pictures of the various abnormal fetuses upset me. So I read a couple of books that were written for pregnant women, not medical students, including *Immaculate Deception* by Suzanne Arms, a passionate attack on the American way of childbirth which argues that many routine hospital practices are psychologically damaging and medically hazardous. In particular, Arms protested the "traditional birth," the euphemism used in opposition to "natural birth." Traditional often means giving birth while lying down, a position demonstrated to be less effective and more dangerous than many others, but convenient for the doctor. An intravenous line is often attached to the arm and an electronic fetal heart monitor strapped to the belly. Traditional almost always means a routine episiotomy, a surgical incision in the perineum to allow the baby's head to emerge without tearing the mother.

In our reproductive medicine course this fall, the issue of home birth came up exactly once, in a "case" for discussion. "BB is a 25-year-old married graduate student . . . ," the case began. BB had a completely normal pregnancy. She showed no unusual symptoms and had no relevant past medical problems. When the pregnancy reached full term, the summary concluded, "no factors have been identified to suggest increased risk." Then, the first question: "Do you think she should choose to deliver at home?"

The doctor leading our discussion section read the question aloud and waited. "No," chorused the class.

"Why not?" asked the doctor.

"Well, there's always the chance of a complication," said one of the students.

Sure enough, after answering the first set of questions, we went on with BB's case, and it turned out that she went two and a half weeks past her due date,

began to show signs of fetal distress, and was ultimately delivered by cesarean after the failure of in-
duced labor. It was clear what the lesson was that BB
was supposed to teach us. It was hard to read the case
without getting the impression that all of these problems were some kind of divine retribution for even
considering a home birth.

In fact, Larry and I eventually decided on a hospital
birth with a doctor whose orientation was clearly against
intervention except where absolutely necessary; he did
not feel that procedures that can help in the event of
complications should be applied across the board. It
pleased me that he volunteered the cesarean and episiotomy figures for his practice, and also that he regarded the issue of what kind of birth we wanted as an
appropriate subject for discussion at our very first
meeting. ("A low-tech birth?" he said, sounding
amused. "You're at Harvard Medical School and you
want a low-tech birth?") He seemed to accept that
there were consumer issues involved in choosing a
doctor—that expectant parents are entitled to an explanation of the doctor's approach early in the pregnancy, when changing doctors is still a reasonable
possibility.

At the beginning of my eighth month, we went to
the first meeting of a prepared-childbirth class spon-
sored by the hospital we had decided to use. I had
great hopes of this class; I was tired of feeling like the
only pregnant person in the world. My medical school
classmates had continued to be extremely kind and
considerate, but as I moved around the medical school
I was beginning to feel like a lone hippopotamus in a
gaggle of geese. I wanted some other people with
whom Larry and I could go over the questions we
discussed endlessly with each other: how do we know
when it's time to leave for the hospital? what is labor

going to *feel* like? what can we do to make it go more easily?

The prepared-childbirth class met in the hospital. At the first meeting, it became clear that its major purpose was to prepare people to be good patients. The teacher was exposing us to various procedures so we would cooperate properly when they were performed on us. Asked whether a given procedure was absolutely necessary, the teacher said that was up to the doctor.

I found a childbirth class that met at a local day-care center; we sat on cushions on the floor, surrounded by toys and children's artwork. Many members of the class were fairly hostile toward the medical profession; once again I was greeted with remarks like "A medical student and you think you want a natural birth? Don't you get thrown out of school for that?" This class was, if anything, designed to teach people how to be "bad patients." The teacher explained the pros and cons of the various interventions, and we discussed under what circumstances we might or might not accept them.

The childbirth classes not only prepared me well for labor but also provided that sense of community I wanted. Yet they also left me feeling pulled between two poles, especially if I went to medical school during the day to discuss deliveries going wrong in one catastrophic way after another ("C-section, C-section!" my discussion section once chanted when the teacher asked what we would do next) and then later to childbirth class in the evening to discuss ways to circumvent unwanted medical procedures. As a student of the medical profession, I know I am being trained to rely heavily on technology, to assume that the risk of acting is almost always preferable to the risk of not acting. I consciously had to fight these attitudes when I thought about giving birth.

*   *   *

In our reproductive medicine course, the emphasis was on the abnormal, the pathological. We learned almost nothing about normal pregnancy; the only thing said about nutrition, for example, was said in passing— that nobody knows how much weight a pregnant woman should gain, but "about twenty-four pounds" is considered good. In contrast, I and the other women in my childbirth class were very concerned with what we ate; we were always exchanging suggestions on how to get through those interminable four glasses of milk a day. We learned nothing in medical school about exercise, though exercise books and classes aimed at pregnant women continue to proliferate—will we, as doctors, be able to give valid advice about diet and exercise during pregnancy? We learned nothing about any of the problems encountered in a normal pregnancy; the only thing said about morning sickness was that it could be controlled with a drug—a drug which, as it happens, many pregnant women are reluctant to take because some studies have linked it to birth defects. We learned nothing about the emotional aspects of pregnancy, nothing about helping women prepare for labor and delivery. In other words, none of my medical school classmates, after the course, would have been capable of answering even the most basic questions about pregnancy asked by the people in my childbirth class. The important issues for future doctors simply did not overlap with the important issues for future parents.

I sat with my classmates in our reproductive medicine course in Amphitheater E at Harvard Medical School and listened to the lecture on the disorders of pregnancy. The professor discussed ectopic pregnancy, toxemia, spontaneous abortion, and major birth defects. I was eight months pregnant. I sat there rubbing my belly, telling my baby, don't worry, you're okay, you're healthy. I sat there wishing that this course would tell us more about normal pregnancy, that after memorizing all the possible disasters, we would be allowed to conclude that pregnancy itself is not a state of disease. But I think most of us, including me, came away from the course with a sense that in fact pregnancy is a deeply dangerous medical condition, that one walks a fine line, avoiding one serious problem after another, to reach the statistically unlikely outcome of a healthy baby and a healthy mother.

I mentioned this to my doctor, explaining that I was tormented by fears of every possible abnormality. "Yes," he said, "normal birth is not honored enough in the curriculum. Most of us doctors are going around looking for pathology and feeling good about ourselves when we find it because that's what we were trained to do. We aren't trained to find joy in a normal pregnancy."

I tried to find joy in my own pregnancy. I am sure that the terrors that sometimes visited me in the middle of the night were no more intense than those that visit most expectant mothers: will the labor go well? will the baby be okay? I probably had more specific fears than many, as I lay awake wondering about atrial septal heart defects or placenta previa and hemorrhage. And perhaps I did worry more than I might once have done, because my faith in the normal had been weakened. I too, in my dark moments, had begun to see healthy development as less than probable, as the highly unlikely avoidance of a million abnormalities. I knew that many of my classmates were worrying with me; I cannot count the number of times I was asked whether I had had an amniocentesis. When I pointed out that we had been taught that amniocentesis is not generally recommended for women under the age of thirty-five, my classmates tended to look worried and mutter something about being *sure*.

The climax came when a young man in my class

asked me, "Have you had all those genetic tests? Like for sickle-cell anemia?"

I looked at him. He is white. I am white. "I'm not in the risk group for sickle-cell," I said gently.

"Yeah, I know," he said, "but if there's even a one-in-a-zillion chance—"

I see all of us, including myself, absorbing the idea that when it comes to tests, technology, interventions, more is better. There was no talk in the reproductive medicine course about the negative aspects of intervention, and the one time a student asked in class about the "appropriateness" of fetal monitoring, the question was cut off with a remark that there was no time to discuss issues of "appropriateness." There was also no time really to discuss techniques for attending women in labor—except as they related to labor emergencies.

I see us absorbing the attitude, here as in other courses, that the kinds of decisions that have to be made are absolutely out of the reach of nonphysicians. The risks of devastating catastrophe are so constant— how can we let patients take chances like this with their lives? Those dangers which can actually be controlled by the patients, the pregnant women—cigarettes, alcohol—are deemphasized. Instead, we are taught to think in terms of medical emergencies. And gradually pregnancy itself begins to sound like a medical emergency in which the pregnant woman, referred to as "the patient," must be carefully guided to a safe delivery, almost in spite of herself. And as we spend more and more time absorbing the vocabulary of medicine, it becomes harder to think about communicating our knowledge to those who lack that vocabulary.

There have been very positive aspects of having the baby while in medical school. For one thing, the anatomy and physiology and embryology I have learned deepened my awe of the miracle going on inside me.

When I looked ahead to the birth, I thought of what we learned about the incredible changeover that takes place during the first minutes of life, about the details of the switch to breathing air, the changes in circulation. I feel that because of what I have learned I appreciated the pregnancy in a way I never could have before, and I am grateful for that appreciation.

Another wonderful thing about having my baby while in medical school was the support and attention from my classmates. Perhaps because having a baby seems a long way off to many of them, there has been some tendency to regard mine as a "class baby." People asked me all the time to promise that I would bring it to lecture; the person who shows the slides offered to dim the lights for a soothing atmosphere if I wanted to nurse in class. My classmates held a baby shower for Larry and me, and presented us with a fabulous assortment of baby items. At the end of the shower, I lay back on the couch with five medical students feeling my abdomen, finding the baby's bottom, the baby's foot.

Our son, Benjamin Orlando, was born on January 28, 1984. Naturally, I would like to be able to say that all our planning and preparing was rewarded with a perfectly smooth, easy labor and delivery, but of course biology doesn't work that way. The experience did provide me with a rather ironic new wrinkle on the whole idea of interventions. Most of the labor was quite ordinary. "You're demonstrating a perfect Friedman labor curve," the doctor said to me at one point, "you must have been studying!" At the end, however, I had great difficulty pushing the baby out. After the pushing stage had gone on for quite a while, I was absolutely exhausted, though the baby was fine; there were no signs of fetal distress and the head was descending steadily. Still, the pushing had gone on much longer than is usual, and I was aware that there were now two doctors and a number of nurses in the birthing room. Suddenly I heard one of the doctors say something about forceps. At that moment, I found a last extra ounce of strength and pushed my baby out. As I lay back with my son wriggling on my stomach, the birthing room suddenly transformed into the most beautiful place on earth, I heard one of the nurses say to another, "You see this all the time with these birthing-room natural-childbirth mothers—you just mention forceps and they get those babies born."

THE CLINICAL YEARS

Why, as a child in the nursery, when her sister had shown a healthy pleasure in tearing her dolls to pieces, had *she* shown an almost morbid one in sewing them up again?

LYTTON STRACHEY,
"Florence Nightingale," in *Eminent Victorians*

WELL, YOU CAN ABSOLUTELY MEMORIZE your textbooks, you can earn a perfect score on every multiple-choice test, but none of that leaves you equipped to take care of patients. Clinical medicine has to be learned as an apprenticeship. And so, armed with your fund of knowledge, you set out into the hospitals. The third and fourth years of medical school were arranged as a series of clinical clerkships (also called rotations). Some were required—three months of general medicine; two of surgery; one each of pediatrics, psychiatry, radiology, neurology, obstetrics, and gynecology; two weeks each of otolaryngology, orthopedics, ophthalmology, dermatology; these were intended to teach basic skills to anyone entering any area of medicine, and also to expose us all to our various career options. Then there was time for clinical electives: advanced courses in an area you were thinking of going into, or just subjects you found interesting, anything from forensic psychiatry to clinical genetics.

What does an "apprentice" do in the hospital? Well, in the more serious clerkships, you take some responsibility for a certain number of patients, "following" them through their time in the hospital, writing notes in their charts, reporting on them to the people above you. You get to play, more or less, the role of doctor to those patients. And then you go and read up on their diseases, and thus add to your fund of knowledge, case by case.

Immediately above you are the interns and residents, the house staff. Interns are in their first year out of medical school, residents in their second or third (or in surgery, which has a longer training period, their fourth or fifth). Senior to the residents there are fellows, doing specialized training in some area (gastroenterology, pulmonary medicine, etc.) and sometimes called in to consult on complex patients. The ward team of interns and residents (and medical students) takes care of the patients from day to day, and is supervised by the attending physician, the senior doctor. At the beginning of the day, the team holds work rounds, catching up on what is going on with each patient, what tests need to be ordered, what changes in management need to be made. The attending later conducts formal teaching sessions, attending rounds, at which particular cases are discussed in detail and medical students, traditionally, are grilled—more or less gently, depending on the attending. The hospital day may include various other kinds of rounds— X-ray rounds, social-service rounds, chief-resident rounds. When I did my surgery clerkship, salesmen from drug companies would sometimes show up with pizza for the doctors, and an announcement would come over the PA system: "Surgical metabolic rounds are beginning in the residents' lounge, immediately."

Aside from rounds, the medical student does more or less whatever doctors in that field do. In surgery, you spend your mornings in the operating room, your afternoons checking incision sites, infections. In general medicine, you draw blood and do spinal taps, you schedule tests and check results. You admit new patients and "work them up," doing whatever kind of exam is appropriate to that particular field, whether it's a full psychiatric history and mental status exam, or a physical exam on a two-month-old. You generally follow the intern's schedule, and the more intense clerkships involve a fair amount of call— staying overnight in the hospital. This can be every other night (surgery) or every third (medicine, pediatrics) or the more benign every fourth (medicine or pediatrics in a different hospital).

The clinical years, especially the third year, are in some ways a very harsh experience. It is frightening to feel yourself very ignorant in a setting where sick people are depending on you for care. It is terrifying to learn on patients how to start an IV. You worry about making a mistake. You worry about hurting someone. On a different level, you worry about making a fool of yourself, about looking stupid on rounds. Your performance in the hospital will affect your future; if you do well, you will have the option of coming back to that program for internship and residency, or else having an enthusiastic evaluation included in your internship letter of recommendation which is sent to other programs. Frequently, medical students care deeply about what will be written in their clerkship evaluations, about who will get an "excellent." Sometimes there is even a highly unpleasant atmosphere of competition between the two or three medical students on a team. There is one-upmanship; one student, for example, was known to read up on his partner's patients, in hopes of outshining that partner in attending rounds the next day.

The other harsh aspect of the clinical years is that the medical student is at the very bottom of a fairly rigid hierarchy. There are often interns and residents who need someone to dump on; they are under a great deal of pressure, they are sometimes treated roughly by senior doctors, they are deprived of sleep—and when they need to kick the proverbial cat, there is the medical student. The experience of always being treated like someone who doesn't matter, of being made to wait constantly, of casually being told to go do this and that, of having your best efforts mocked or your ignorance held up for all to see—this can make you desperately resentful. "For this I'm paying a thousand dollars a month," I used to hiss through clenched teeth.

I have described all this to try to give some context to the bitterness which comes through in a number of the pieces that follow. Although I learned an enormous amount in my clinical clerkships, I also wasted a fair amount of time, and it was not time I spared gladly; when you have been in the hospital for over thirty-six hours straight, you do not necessarily want to sit and listen to an attending ramble on about how much better everything was back when he was an intern. Or listen to some resident discourse on the way the fellows tried to push him around, and what he said to them. One of the sad effects of my clinical training was that I think I generally became a more impatient, unpleasant person. Time was precious, sleep was often insufficient, and in the interests of my evaluations, I had to treat all kinds of turkeys with profound respect. Well, you see what I mean.

My clinical clerkships did what they were supposed to do. They taught me to survive in the hospital, to take care of my patients, find out what I didn't know. I learned the anatomy and physiology of a hospital, the logic of its complex organization. And I learned the cast of characters, the language, the rhythms. I became someone who can move, without any particular conscious effort, into that other world. It is hard to remember what it was like to be so achingly self-conscious, back at the beginning, to feel so out of place. The hospital was an alien and somewhat hostile environment, and now it is my territory.

The First Time

There is a first time for everything, of course. For the medical student, back at the very beginning of the long path through medical training, there are terrifying first times for each of any number of small everyday hospital procedures. I think of drawing blood, the most common of these procedures, as a metaphor for much of what we do in the hospital: it involves the direct violation of the body's integrity, the causing of pain, and the removal of ordinarily hidden body substance for examination in the bright light of a microscope.

You wrap the tourniquet around the patient's arm and hope the veins bulge slightly into view. You swab with alcohol. You slide the needle in, as gently as you can, and pull back on the plunger, hoping to see blood rising into the syringe.

For the past two years I have been a medical student, studying my textbooks, sitting in lectures, looking through microscopes at slides, dissecting a cadaver. This summer I did my first "clinical clerkship," working in the hospital. I "followed" a certain number of patients, seeing them every day, doing my best to understand everything that happened to them, reading up on their medical problems. I also did a good deal of what we call "scut," those little jobs, like drawing blood, which inevitably fall down the chain of command to land in the medical student's lap.

And so for the first time I found myself standing next to a sick person with a hypodermic in my hand, while from across the bed an intern said to me, "Okay, see if you can locate a vein."

Patients were remarkably cooperative, which was partially the magic of the white coat; wear it and everyone assumes you know what you're doing, no matter how obviously you may be fumbling. Also, the idea of doctors-in-training is very frightening; many patients don't like to face the fact that the people making decisions about their health may be in some sense just beginners.

The aphorism is "See one, do one, teach one." In theory, someone senior to you should walk you through each procedure slowly the first time, leaving you confident and ready to do it on your own the next time.

"With blood gases, for me it's more like see three, try four, miss them all," said a friend of mine. Drawing blood gases means getting blood from the artery instead of the vein. The artery is harder to find than the vein, and the process can be excruciating for the patient—especially if you miss the artery the first couple of times. There was a patient on the ward where I worked for my first few weeks this summer who finally rebelled. We marched in one morning on rounds, the whole crowd of us, one resident, two interns, two medical students. The resident asked the patient how she was doing, listened to her chest, and said to me, "Perri, let's get another blood gas on her."

"Oh no," said the patient, "I'm not letting her near me. She tried the other day."

"Okay," said the resident, smiling at my apologetic grimace, pointing to the other medical student. "How about him? He's very good."

"Oh, no he's not!" said the patient. "He tried too the other day. I'm not letting either of them near me."

She pointed to one of the interns. "You do it, you have a light touch."

But most patients didn't object, and so I made my way through the summer, drawing blood from veins and arteries as the occasion required, but also putting a tube up someone's nose and down into his stomach for the first time, starting an intravenous line for the first time, and moving on to procedures which are more complex and also genuinely more dangerous—like my first spinal tap. There has to be a first time for everything.

There is also the patient's first time, of course. And just as drawing blood, a procedure completely straight-forward and routine to the hospital blood technician, can be terrifying and extremely complex to the beginning medical student, it is important to remember that procedures and exams which for some patients are not at all traumatic can be tremendously difficult and painful for other patients.

One night early in the summer the intern I was working with asked me to assist her in doing a pelvic exam. The patient was a woman who had come to the hospital because she was feeling a little weak, and who had been discovered to have cancer in several places, cancer which looked metastatic. The problem then was to locate the primary site of her cancer, and the pelvic exam was the first in a series of attempts. The intern, a woman a year or so older than I, actually performed the pelvic; all I did was hold a flashlight—and the patient's hand. She was a woman in her seventies with a sweet face and a gentle smile and, just to complete the picture, an armful of fuzzy knitting. We put her knitting on the bedside table, and, because we had no examining table with stirrups, we propped her up in bed on a bedpan for the exam.

"You probably had one of these exams when you had children," said the intern.

"Oh, no," said the patient, smiling at us, "why, I've never even been married."

"Oh, okay," said the intern. "Well, I want you to know that Perri and I have both had this done to us, and nobody really likes having it done, but we'll be as quick as we can."

And so we did the pelvic, with the poor lady crying out in pain and surprise, because this was something she was not expecting, was not prepared for. In a certain sense this exam, so routine for most women, was an initiation for this woman into a part of her life which will be full of invasive tests, of pain she will be told is necessary, a part of her life she was not expecting. Our white-coated authority offered her no comfort; wanting to help her, we found ourselves reaching for some element of solidarity, reminding her that we had been patients too, that all three of us had a common anatomy.

And in the end, perhaps that is the lesson that comes with experience in those things I do that cause patients pain: as I become a little more experienced, a little more sure of myself, I become less anxious to retreat behind the barrier of professionalism. Even with drawing blood—the first few times I did it, I was terrified the patient would see how nervous I was and would guess why. "You'll just feel a little stick," I would say cheerfully, trying desperately to find the vein. By now, reasonably sure that I can find the vein if it's there to be found, I am much less afraid to let the patient see if I am puzzled or unsure. "This will hurt a little, but I'll do it as quickly as I can," I say. Perhaps there is an implicit apology in my attitude, and that does not seem to me to be such a bad thing, because surely there ought to be some acknowledgment in such a situation that however necessary the pain may be, I am not the one who has to bear it.

Crying in the Hospital

It had been a long and difficult night in the hospital, I had gotten only two hours of sleep, and toward morning, a young patient had died of cancer. I was sitting in the nurses' coffee room, staring into space, when the intern, who had had no sleep at all, who had been responsible for everything on the ward, came in and found me.

"Are you okay?" he asked, and I promptly burst into tears.

And then I lied. I told the intern that I was crying for the young woman who had died, whose parents were sitting by her bed, dazed and saddened by the ending of a long and terrible ordeal. I said I was crying for the patient, and for her parents, but I knew that in large part I was crying for myself. I was crying because I hadn't slept much, and because I had a long day in front of me in which I would be put on the spot and have my ignorance revealed again and again, a day throughout which I would feel tired and sick and heavy-headed and inadequate. And also, of course, because a young woman had died. It was embarrassing enough to be crying in front of the intern; the least I could do was pretend my motives were purely sympathetic and altruistic, rather than substantially mixed with self-pity.

The prospect of crying in the hospital haunts many women I meet, medical students like me, and interns as well. It seems to hover on the edge of our minds as something we are likely to do, something we must not do because it will confirm all the most clichéd objections to women as doctors. Crying will compromise our professionalism as well as our strength. Actually, before I started my clinical clerkship in the hospital, it never occurred to me to think of myself as someone who cried in public.

But it turned out that I cried frequently and helplessly in the hospital. My very first week there, I discovered that there was one particular room I could not enter on morning rounds without tears starting to slide down my face. The rooms were decorated with large prints of impressionist paintings, and that particular room had a Mary Cassatt painting, a woman holding a child. I had suddenly found myself working over a hundred hours a week, spending every third night in the hospital, and I missed my baby badly. I simply could not look at that painting.

I cried for the patients. I cried after a man talked to me for fifteen minutes about what a vigorous, lively, intelligent person his wife had been before her stroke, and then took my hand, called me "Doctor," and begged me to hold out some hope that she would be that way again.

I cried because I forgot to do things. I cried because I didn't know how to do things. I cried because I did things, only to find out they were unnecessary. In fact, looking back on those first couple of weeks in the hospital, it seems to me I was always ducking into bathrooms to sniffle into paper towels and splash cold water on my face. I cried, but I took great care not to be seen at it.

I have come to realize that I was not the only one crying. A friend told me about crying because a patient was dying and she could do nothing to help and everyone kept saying it was a "fascinating case." An intern told me about crying because one night when she was swamped she asked a more senior doctor for help, only to be told off the next day because asking for help was a confession of "weakness." We all cry, perhaps, because we are in a harsh environment, an environment that offers us little comfort, and in which we frequently find ourselves unable to offer comfort to others.

I brought up the subject with a couple of male students. No, they said, of course they got upset, and frustrated, and unhappy, but it hadn't gotten so bad they actually *cried*. This may simply reflect the much-remarked-on truth that men are slower to tears than women in this society, and it may also suggest that the hospital is still a very male environment, the medical hierarchy created by generations of male doctors—maybe it all seems a little more comfortable to male students. Or again, maybe they were lying; maybe they were just too ashamed of those tearful moments in the bathroom and the weakness they implied.

I cried so easily last summer because some of my protection was stripped away. Working in the hospital, even as a student with very limited responsibility, I was constantly on the line. Did you do this? Why not? What would have been the right thing to do? What are the possible consequences of what you didn't do? Precisely because I was a student, I was questioned regularly by any number of people, some of whom were under tremendous pressure themselves, and not inclined to make allowances for my greenness. The steady tension, the fear of making a mistake, and the mistakes which inevitably do get made can raise the emotional pitch much too high for comfort. In addition, I was sleep-deprived, and deprived of any time for my family or friends, for anything that might have mitigated the intensity. And finally, the hospital is a place where all sorts of emotions are visible. I saw people mourning and people screaming with pain, people crying with terror and people dying. It's hard to say exactly what effect it has, this everyday drama and melo-drama, but perhaps it led me to exaggerate my emo-tional responses to the tiny dramas of my own life: will I get three hours of sleep tonight or only two? will I remember what I read last night about heart disease when they quiz me this morning?

It is easy to lose your sense of proportion in the hospital. In fact, it is hard to know what "proportion" means in a place where people are struggling for their lives, or living with tremendous pain. The medical student, like the intern, tries to maintain both balance and compassion on a schedule that allows for little rest and no relief. And frequently she runs the risk of being overwhelmed, by sorrow for others, by tired hopelessness about her own competence, or by help-less anger at doctors whose idea of teaching involves constant tests of strength and occasional humiliation.

I wish I had been telling the whole truth when I said I was crying for the patient who died that night. I can accept my own compassion much more easily than I can accept the mixture of disorientation, inadequacy, and self-pity which was actually behind most of my crying in the hospital. And yet, I suppose, accepting those less than nobly sensitive motives is also a neces-sary step toward acknowledging my own human limi-tations. Those limitations, after all, even in this age of technological health care, are also in some sense the limitations of the medical profession, whether or not it cares to admit them.

Camels, Zebras, and Fascinomas

Morning rounds in the hospital. The interns and the resident and the medical students are crowded into a little room littered with discarded white coats and texts with titles like *Heart Disease Made Simple*. One of the interns is asleep sitting up. Presiding is the attending physician, the senior doctor present, whose job it is to supervise patient care and also to teach the junior members of the team. You, the medical student who was on call last night, are finishing your presentation. You have told the story of the patient you admitted, his history, his physical exam.

"All right, then," says the attending, "the patient has dysphagia, he feels that food sticks in his throat. What's the differential diagnosis of dysphagia?"

This is your moment, the moment for whose sake you gave up your precious hour of sleep last night to sit over a textbook in the hospital library. Surreptitiously, you look down at your notes. You clear your throat. You try to appear as though this sort of information is always on the tip of your tongue. Quickly, you run through some of the more prominent possibilities—muscle disorders, tumors, benign strictures of the esophagus with their various causes. If you're feeling flashy, you list possible diagnoses on the blackboard while the other students look at you with hatred and a second intern goes to sleep. Finally, you get to the really exciting stuff, the *neat* diseases. "Rabies can cause dysphagia," you say happily. "So can vascular compression by aortic aneurysm!" The attending and the resident exchange glances. "Typical medical student," one of them says, patronizingly but fondly. "Really only wants to talk about the zebras."

Peculiar animals roam the halls of medical schools. At Harvard, for example, we get "camels," printed lecture notes for all our courses. "Camel" is presumably a reference to the old line that a camel is a horse created by a committee—our lecture notes, like our courses, are generally group projects. The committee metaphor was often brought home forcefully when I found myself reading through my camel for the first time the night before an exam, wondering desperately how all the pieces fit together to form a single credible beast.

And then there are "zebras"; this term comes from a rather rueful joke. The idea is that when a normal person (not a medical student or doctor) hears hoofbeats, the first thought that comes to mind is "Horse." But a medical student hears hoofbeats and immediately thinks "Zebra!" Medical students, the cliché goes, think first about the rare, unlikely diagnosis, are uninterested in common medical problems. The medical student not only expects those hoofbeats to be a zebra's, but is actually disappointed to see no exotic black and white stripes, just a plain old horse. And the fact is, the appeal of the rare and dramatic disease is built right into medical training, and the dream of someday lassoing a zebra continues to titillate many of those more advanced people who smile patronizingly at the medical student's crude reflexes.

The goal, of course, isn't to collect oddities but to help people. We sometimes joke about the way we all wrote on our medical school application essays, "I want to become a doctor because I want to help people in need, blah, blah, blah, rewarding, blah, blah,

blah." Like any other subculture, medicine develops
its own internal systems of values, its own hierarchies
of prestige and power. And these don't necessarily
have anything to do with helping patients. That student making the presentation on morning rounds isn't
going to get any brownie points for "sincerity of desire
to help patient." It's time for some academic fire-
works. You bring up all the one-in-a-million possibilities, diagnoses that don't fit this particular patient at
all, and then you smile and say smugly, "Included for
completeness."

Especially at a place like Harvard, there is a subtle
(and sometimes not so subtle) message that everyday
ordinary medicine, the kind you see at every little
"community hospital" (said condescendingly), is just
not very interesting or very exciting—or as we sometimes say, not very glamorous or very sexy. We don't
mean glamorous in the young-TV-doctor-in-white sense,
we mean a more particular glitter. The "top medical
schools" tend to push people toward specialization
and research. Our lecturers used to say to us, maybe
one of you will be the one to figure out this problem.
Or sometimes they just said, you people will be on the
frontiers of medicine, the cutting edge. And our class
would squirm a little, and maybe even hiss a little,
uncomfortably aware that there was something odd
about making that assumption about a group of people
who happened to get past the admissions committee
(". . . blah, blah, help people, blah, blah, rewarding
. . ."). In fact, however, the training does push you in
particular directions, does shape your goals, and your
attitudes as well.

Biomedical research on rare and peculiar diseases
has contributed a great deal to the understanding of
disease and to the care of patients, even patients with
more common problems. But if the general attitude is
that rare diseases are somehow the real "prizes" in the

grab bag of clinical medicine, then students may stop
caring so much about more mundane medical problems, or at least may give less credit to those who
concentrate on them. And the condescension that the
medical student feels toward people who devote themselves to the study of what we call "bread-and-butter
medicine" may not completely disappear as that student grows older and (one hopes) wiser. Academic
medicine is a prestige-conscious world, and some people have trouble getting funding for their work. Bread-
and-butter medicine isn't necessarily the path to
professional advancement in this world; it sometimes
seems that brownie points are awarded in a fashion
rather parallel to that facing the student on rounds.

So back to the medical student, the eager initiate
into the prejudices and rituals of the profession, in
whom its subtle emphases may be most clunkingly
apparent. The medical student's fondness for zebras,
for wildly unlikely diagnoses, is gently (or ungently)
mocked when it gets out of hand—but it's also an
indicator of prejudices shared by senior people, who
express them in a much more veiled and acceptable
manner. I remember once suggesting, "Malaria would
also fit his symptoms, wouldn't it?" about a patient
who the team thought had flu. And I remember my
tiny ignoble *hope* that the patient would in fact turn
out to have malaria (he didn't), that my zebra would,
so to speak, come home to roost. I imagined the other
team members saying, "Actually, the medical student
made the diagnosis. A real fascinoma. Great case."

"Fascinoma" is one of those hospital words. *Oma,*
of course, means tumor, but "fascinoma" is used to
mean any disease remarkable chiefly for its fascination
value. One-of-a-kind diseases, diseases you'll never
see again, diseases unusual in this age or in this country, diseases that are for one reason or another very

difficult to diagnose are fascinomas. They are also "great cases," a term that is used all the time, ostensibly to mean "cases we can all learn a lot from." Medical students in the hospital compete for these patients: "Great case coming in this morning, might be Wegener's granulomatosis. Definite medical student case—who wants it?" You all jump. Even if you're not really in the mood for another great case, you still don't want people to think you're less than gung ho. And for the rest of the time the patient is in the hospital, everyone who comes around to consult will say, "Is this your patient? Great case." They'll go on saying it even if the patient is dying, which can be disturbing to a medical student who has come to see the patient as something more than a teaching exercise. A great case is a great case, even when it's dying.

So there you are on rounds, talking about that patient with dysphagia. You list the diagnoses. You get told not to waste your time on the zebras: the patient has either a benign stricture or a malignancy. The rest of morning rounds is devoted to sodium disturbances, your attending's special field of interest. This patient, the one with the dysphagia, happens to have a slightly high but still normal sodium level. Your attending wants to know what the possible diagnoses would be if the level were a little higher. Like a fool, you didn't read up on this last night; instead, you're stuffed to the gills with hastily memorized facts about esophageal diseases, not to mention rabies and aortic aneurysms. It isn't one of your more distinguished performances. Even the resident falls asleep.

And then your luck changes. The patient's esophagus turns out to be completely free of tumor or stricture. In fact, the patient has a rare, irreversible, progressive neurological disease, which will make it necessary for him to eat through a tube surgically implanted in his stomach, a disease that will eventually kill him. From rather unpromising beginnings, you have got yourself a real fascinoma.

Learning the Language

"Mrs. Tolstoy is your basic LOL in NAD, admitted for a soft rule-out MI," the intern announces. I scribble that on my patient list. In other words, Mrs. Tolstoy is a Little Old Lady in No Apparent Distress who is in the hospital to make sure she hasn't had a heart attack (rule out a Myocardial Infarction). And we think it's unlikely that she has had a heart attack (a *soft* rule-out).

If I learned nothing else during my first three months of working in the hospital as a medical student, I learned endless jargon and abbreviations. I started out in a state of primeval innocence, in which I didn't even know that "s̄ CP, SOB, N/V" meant "without chest pain, shortness of breath, or nausea and vomiting." By the end I took the abbreviations so much for granted that I would complain to my mother the English professor, "And can you believe I had to put down *three* NG tubes last night?"

"You'll have to tell me what an NG tube is if you want me to sympathize properly," my mother said. NG, nasogastric—isn't it obvious?

I picked up not only the specific expressions but also the patterns of speech and the grammatical conventions; for example, you never say that a patient's blood pressure fell or that his cardiac enzymes rose. Instead, the patient is always the subject of the verb: "He dropped his pressure." "He bumped his enzymes." This sort of construction probably reflects the profound irritation of the intern when the nurses come in the middle of the night to say that Mr. Dickinson has disturbingly low blood pressure. "Oh, he's gonna hurt me bad tonight," the intern might say, inevitably angry at Mr. Dickinson for dropping his pressure and creating a problem.

When chemotherapy fails to cure Mrs. Bacon's cancer, what we say is, "Mrs. Bacon failed chemotherapy."

"Well, we've already had one hit today, and we're up next, but at least we've got mostly stable players on our team." This means that our team (group of doctors and medical students) has already gotten one new admission today, and it is our turn again, so we'll get whoever is admitted next in emergency, but at least most of the patients we already have are fairly stable, that is, unlikely to drop their pressures or in any other way get suddenly sicker and hurt us bad. Baseball metaphor is pervasive. A no-hitter is a night without any new admissions. A player is always a patient—a nitrate player is a patient on nitrates, a unit player is a patient in the intensive care unit, and so on, until you reach the terminal player.

It is interesting to consider what it means to be winning, or doing well, in this perennial baseball game. When the intern hangs up the phone and announces, "I got a hit," that is not cause for congratulations. The team is not scoring points; rather, it is getting hit, being bombarded with new patients. The object of the game from the point of view of the doctors, considering the players for whom they are already responsible, is to get as few new hits as possible.

This special language contributes to a sense of closeness and professional spirit among people who are under a great deal of stress. As a medical student, I found it exciting to discover that I'd finally cracked the code, that I could understand what doctors said and wrote, and could use the same formulations myself. Some people seem to become enamored of the jargon for its own sake, perhaps because they are so deeply thrilled with the idea of medicine, with the idea of themselves as doctors.

I knew a medical student who was referred to by the interns on the team as Mr. Eponym because he was so infatuated with eponymous terminology, the more obscure the better. He never said "capillary pulsations" if he could say "Quincke's pulses." He would lovingly tell over the multinamed syndromes—Wolff-Parkinson-White, Lown-Ganong-Levine, Schönlein-Henoch—until the temptation to suggest Schleswig-Holstein or Stevenson-Kefauver or Baskin-Robbins became irresistible to his less reverent colleagues.

And there is the jargon that you don't ever want to hear yourself using. You know that your training is changing you, but there are certain changes you think would be going a little too far.

The resident was describing a man with devastating terminal pancreatic cancer. "Basically he's CTD," the resident concluded. I reminded myself that I had resolved not to be shy about asking when I didn't understand things. "CTD?" I asked timidly.

The resident smirked at me. "Circling The Drain."

The images are vivid and terrible. "What happened to Mrs. Melville?"

"Oh, she boxed last night." To box is to die, of course.

Then there are the more pompous locutions that can make the beginning medical student nervous about the effects of medical training. A friend of mine was told by his resident, "A pregnant woman with sickle-cell represents a failure of genetic counseling."

Mr. Eponym, who tried hard to talk like the doctors, once explained to me, "An infant is basically a brainstem preparation." The term "brainstem preparation," as used in neurological research, refers to an animal whose higher brain functions have been destroyed so that only the most primitive reflexes remain, like the sucking reflex, the startle reflex, and the rooting reflex.

And yet at other times the harshness dissipates into a strangely elusive euphemism. "As you know, this is a not entirely benign procedure," some doctor will say, and that will be understood to imply agony, risk of complications, and maybe even a significant mortality rate.

The more extreme forms aside, one most important function of medical jargon is to help doctors maintain some distance from their patients. By reformulating a patient's pain and problems into a language that the patient doesn't even speak, I suppose we are in some sense taking those pains and problems under our jurisdiction and also reducing their emotional impact. This linguistic separation between doctors and patients allows conversations to go on at the bedside that are unintelligible to the patient. "Naturally, we're worried about adeno-CA," the intern can say to the medical student, and lung cancer need never be mentioned.

I learned a new language this past summer. At times it thrills me to hear myself using it. It enables me to understand my colleagues, to communicate effectively in the hospital. Yet I am uncomfortably aware that I will never again notice the peculiarities and even atrocities of medical language as keenly as I did this summer. There may be specific expressions I manage to avoid, but even as I remark them, promising myself I will never use them, I find that this language is becoming my professional speech. It no longer sounds strange in my ears—or coming from my mouth. And I am afraid that as with any new language, to use it properly you must absorb not only the vocabulary but also the structure, the logic, the attitudes. At first you may notice these new and alien assumptions every time you put together a sentence, but with time and increased fluency you stop being aware of them at all. And as you lose that awareness, for better or for worse, you move closer and closer to being a doctor instead of just talking like one.

Macho

Purely by coincidence, our team has four women and one man. The two interns and the two medical students are female, and the resident, who leads the team, is male. We are clattering up the stairs one morning in approved hospital fashion, conveying by our purposeful demeanor: out of the way, doctors coming, decisions to make, lives to save. (In fact, what we are actually trying to do is to rush through morning rounds in time to get to breakfast before the cafeteria stops serving hot food, but never mind that now.) We barrel through the door into the intensive care unit, and some other resident, standing by, announces, "Here comes The A-Team." Immediately our resident swings around to respond to some undertone he has detected:

"Are you saying my team is weak? Huh? You saying my team is weak?"

We continue on our rounds, the resident occasionally prompting one of the interns, "You should be pushing me out of the way, you know. Go on, push me out of the way." He means that since she is on call that day, she should be first through every door, first to lay hands on every patient.

My fellow medical student and I trail along in the rear, a position that accurately reflects our place in the hierarchy and also my energy level (this is, after all, 7:00 A.M.). She whispers to me, "Straighten your back! Suck in your stomach! This is war!" And as we start to clatter down the stairs to breakfast, our morning mission successfully accomplished, she and I are both singing under our breaths, "Macho macho doc, I wanna be a macho doc. . . ."

Macho in medicine can mean a number of things. Everyone knows it's out there as a style, either an ideal or an object of ridicule. You hear echoes of it in the highest praise one can receive in the hospital, "Strong work," which may be said to an intern who got a very sick patient through the night or to a medical student who successfully fielded some obscure questions on rounds. And the all-purpose term of disparagement is "Weak." They're being really weak down in the emergency room tonight, admitting people who could just as well be sent home. Dr. So-and-so is being weak with that patient—why doesn't he just tell him he *has* to have the surgery? You were pretty weak this morning when they were asking you about rheumatic heart disease—better read up on it.

Macho can refer to your willingness to get tough with your patients, to keep them from pushing you around. It can refer to your eagerness to do invasive procedures—"The hell with radiology, I wanna go for the biopsy." Talk like that and they'll call you a cowboy, and generally mean it as a compliment. Macho can mean territoriality: certain doctors resent calling in expert consultations and, when they finally have to, await the recommendations with truculent eagerness to disregard them. "These are *our* patients and *we* make all the decisions," I heard over and over from one resident I worked under. The essence of macho, any kind of macho, after all, is that life is a perpetual contest. You must not let others intrude on your stamping grounds. You must not let anyone tell you what to do. And of course, the most basic macho fear is the fear of being laughed at; whatever you do, you must not let anyone mock you—or your team.

A medical student once said to me when I teased him about not being able to work the Addressograph machine after six weeks in the hospital, "That's secretarial work. I can draw a blood gas blindfolded, from thirty feet away!"

Life in the hospital is full of opportunities to prove yourself, if you want to look at it that way. "I want you guys to be able to get blood from a stone," announced our new resident on his first day as our leader. The "guys," the other female medical student and I, must have looked a little dubious, because he continued, "Okay, it may mean the patient gets stuck a few extra times, but I don't want you giving up just because of that." And sure enough, when I came to tell him that I had stuck one particular woman six times without success, and could he please come show me where he thought a decent vein might be, he sent me back in to try her ankles. "Blood from a stone!" he called after me, and when I finally got a tube of this unfortunate woman's blood, he patted me on the back and said, "Strong work."

If we are at war, then who is the enemy? Rightly the enemy is disease, and even if that is not your favorite metaphor, it is a rather common way to think of medicine: we are combating these deadly processes for the bodies of our patients. They become battlefields, lying there passively in bed while the evil armies of pathology and the resplendent forces of modern medicine fight it out. Still, there are very good doctors who seem to think that way, who take disease as a personal enemy and battle it with fury and dedication. The real problem arises because all too often the patient comes to personify the disease, and somehow the patient becomes the enemy.

We don't say, or think, "Mrs. Hawthorne's cancer is making her sicker." We say, "Mrs. Hawthorne's crumping on me," and Mrs. Hawthorne represents the challenge we cannot meet, the disease we cannot cure. And instead of hating her cancer, it's not hard to start hating Mrs. Hawthorne—especially if she has an irritating personality, and most especially of all if she somehow seems to be blaming us. That is, if every day the doctor sees the challenge again in the patient's eye, hears it in the patient's voice: "You can't do anything for me, can you, despite all the tests and all the medicines?"

The patient may want the doctor to continue fighting, may even take renewed hope as new therapies are instituted, but the doctor, knowing them to be essentially futile, may become angrier and angrier. When the disease has essentially won and the patient continues to present the challenge, the macho doctor is left with no appropriate response. He cannot sidestep the challenge by offering comfort rather than combat, because comfort is not in his repertoire. And unable to do battle against the disease to any real effect, he may feel almost ready to battle the patient.

I have been talking as if macho medicine is a male preserve, and to a large extent that's true. Certainly there are some female doctors who end up being fairly macho and, much more important, many men who are not macho at all. Some of the gentlest, most reasonable doctors I worked with were male, good teachers and superb healers. But there are also many macho docs, and certainly it is pervasive as a style in the hospital. I don't believe that would be the case if the majority of doctors up to now had been female, and perhaps it will change over time as more women become doctors. The tradition of medical training is partly a tradition of hazing, boot camp, basic training. New buzzwords are now being muttered, like "nurturing" or "supportive," but there are many doctors riding the range out there to whom you wouldn't dare mutter any such words.

"Sup-por-tive," you can almost hear The Duke drawl as the doctor looks down at the newest sissy in town. At which point you tuck your hypodermic needle back into its holster and march, on the double, back into that pesky varmint's room to let him know who's boss in this here hospital.

Tempos

Many of my medical school classmates are the children of doctors. Maybe they grew up understanding such concepts as "on call," "radiology," "attending," and "intern." I, on the other hand, grew up related to no doctors, and like everyone else in America, I watched medical shows on television, with their heroism, their crisp decision ("Scalpel!"), and above all, their neat and symmetrical rhythms. When I started to think about going to medical school, I probably still cherished the notion somewhere that the tempo of a doctor's life was a tempo of tidy one-hour segments with intriguing beginnings, dramatic complications, and satisfying resolutions. In short, I knew as much about the tempo of a doctor's life as I did about a secret agent's—and I was a devoted watcher of *Mission Impossible*. (And I also knew, of course, that both doctors and secret agents were extremely good-looking—but that's another kettle of movie stars.)

And I must say that I got through most of the first two years of medical school without being brought up against most of these issues of tempo. Along with my classmates, I studied the basic sciences, and then pathophysiology, and sometimes when we talked about medicine we discussed large personal questions like Am I Truly Interested in Cardiovascular Pathophysiology, or Are My Hands Skillful Enough for Me to Think of Surgery, or even larger questions like Is Medicine Too

Dehumanized. But mostly we were students, taking courses, and of course we were professionals when it came to multiple-choice tests, and it was reassuring to see them coming round every month or so—but what does that have to do with being a doctor? (Well, quite a bit, it turns out; you can't be a doctor without taking some of the longest and trickiest multiple-choice tests ever dreamed up by a power-mad computer—but that's another kettle of No. 2 pencils.)

And then, finally, in the third and fourth years, you get out into the hospitals and begin seeing patients, and also, of course, seeing doctors, in vivo. And the questions that begin to occur to you then are smaller in scale but infinitely more personal, and very often they are questions of tempo. How do I want to live my life is a very large issue, but God, as usual, is in the details.

Do I want to work with *very* sick patients? How many hours a day do I want to spend in a darkened room? How do I feel about touching and examining bodies? How much drama can I stomach? Do I like making split-second decisions? How much power do I want? Do I yearn to be in a lab?

And the other questions that begin to surface, a little shamefacedly, in the last two years of medical school. Do I want to spend years of my life working all night every third (or every second, or every fourth) night? How early can I stand to get up in the morning? (And then there are the questions you don't dare ask aloud, either because they're too cosmic or else because they're too trivial: what if I never learn how to distinguish heart sounds? how can I survive on hospital cafeteria food? But that's another kettle of vending machines.)

So what you have in the third and fourth years is a veritable smorgasbord of the medical profession, as you dip for a month or two into all the different fields.

Or, to use a different metaphor, you get to try out one tempo and then another, trying to imagine which one will best suit your personality, your fantasies, your life.

There is the profoundly dominant tempo of internal medicine, the slow, talky pace of the morning, rounds and rounds and rounds, the occasional tension of the rapid back-and-forth, the long rhythmic drones of monologue, and then the increasing urgency as the day moves on and any number of separate themes, each with its own particular pattern, blend in alternating harmonies and disharmonies. And the nights, too, with their own peculiar lulls and sudden outbreaks of insane energy, crashes, and confusion. It's easy to get swept away in it, intoxicated by the complexity, and stare out at the world wondering how other people live.

And then consider radiology, days in the dark, staring hard, straight ahead, and trying desperately to learn to see; long silences in which you know there's *something* going on, if only you could perceive it, and then the discursive soliloquies which also build to controversy, but there's a rhythm here of set, specific problems posed, answered, and then the story moves on.

Or psychiatry, where the single voices can be distinguished, and you start to detect amazing subtleties in tone and shading, and the whole thing takes you suddenly into moments of introspection quite unlike anything you've come across so far, as you begin to worry consciously about how you're affected by what you're hearing and seeing. There's a jumpy, tense feel to the rhythm here at times, a wildness being held in check, and sometimes it bursts through and you can hear it being taken over, calmed, subdued.

And then, well, for drama you can't beat surgery. It takes you into a tempo where all nonessentials are speeded up—you dimly recognize the echo of rounds from medicine, as they zip past you triple-time, and lead on into a ritual dance of transformation, getting ready, passing into a new and brightly lit environment where the real business of the day takes place. There is clarity and also rigid hierarchy in this pattern; the dominant voices set the rhythm. And there is also of course the drama of the unexpected, tremendous pressure and complexity and the sense that small mistakes will shatter the pattern into chaos. And then, like medicine, the nights have their own quality, the individual themes that build to hopeful bright resolutions, and the inexorable degenerations into chaos or limbo.

Background noise of crying babies: pediatrics provides its own specific variants on much of what you've seen elsewhere. Each separate story is accompanied by anxious guardians, providing you with counterpoints of questions, fears, and also support. Your overall approach is somewhat different; you find yourself capering and manufacturing lighthearted little trills ("Is that a bird in your ear?") to divert attention from the major work to be accomplished. And the dwindling disasters, when they come, are the worst of all.

And so it goes on, and of course you have no way, really, of knowing what it would be like to live with any of these tempos for years and years. And there are so many you've never been exposed to, so many different kinds of lives led by doctors. The variety defies all your best attempts at sorting out the different variables. So you go on your instincts, and in the third year you begin to hear students say, sometimes with wonder as if they were surprised at themselves:

"I really need a field where I just don't have too much actual contact with patients. I always thought that was the whole point, but it turns out to be the part I don't like."

"I just don't want to work with hospitalized people; I loved the emergency room."

"I always space out as soon as I get into the OR."

"I always space out on rounds."

"It's more satisfying to be there at the major crises in people's lives; I just can't get into all the little every-day things."

And so, despite your efforts to rise above it all, to cram yourself full of medical knowledge and ignore your inconvenient personality, you find yourself in-volved in (shudder) self-discovery. You choose your tempo, or your tempo chooses you, and if you wait for the messages from your sponsor to come break up the day, you may be disappointed. (Or maybe not, if the drug company representatives are around, but that's another kettle of complimentary penlights.)

The Scrubbed
and the Unscrubbed

"So what are you doing in medical school now?"

"Surgery."

"Really, no kidding? You actually *do* surgery?"

"Well, not exactly." [Nonchalant, elaborately casual.] "I just stitch people up, sometimes I get to cut them open."

People are fascinated to hear that you are spending your days in surgery. They want to know, what does it feel like to cut into someone? what does it feel like to sew up skin? Either that, or they don't want to hear anything about it at all, and if you start on one of your surgery stories ("So, we have this guy on the table, and then it turns out no one knows which kidney it is . . ."), they beg you, not at the dinner table, please.

"Is it really weird? Do you feel like you're going to faint?"

"You mean in the OR?" [Ostentatious politeness.] "Sorry, I mean the operating room. Nah, that's fun, really."

Traditionally, in the OR, the medical student holds the retractor. This is the bottom of the totem pole; you stand there and hold onto a specialized hook, pulling the hole (in the chest or the stomach or the neck or wherever) open wider so that the important people, that is, the surgeons, can see what they're doing. You stand frozen in position, holding the retractor as still as possible, torn between a desire not to cause unwanted vibrations and a suspicion that your retractor is no longer necessary and they have forgotten all about you, as your muscles knot and your foot goes to sleep and your nose, under the surgical mask, itches.

And you get asked questions. The surgeon turns to you from time to time (and you are by no means delighted by this evidence that you have not in fact been forgotten) to ask, "Now, what nerves should I be worrying about here?" or "Can you name the layers of muscle I'm slicing through?" The best question I was ever asked in the OR, actually, was, "Do you know 'The Masochism Tango'?" Fortunately, I was brought up on Tom Lehrer songs, and so I was able to make a good impression by reciting a line or two. Even more fortunately, the surgeon did not ask me to sing it, since I am completely tone-deaf. He was too eager to sing it himself, and sing it he did, as he operated:

> *Take your cigarette from its holder*
> *And burn your initials in my shoulder.* . . .

"You really sew people up? Like wounds?"

"Well, wounds, of course. But mostly I do some of the big surgical incisions—you know, like sewing up someone's stomach." [Carefree lightness.] "But a lot of times nowadays they just use staples to close people up, so I don't get to do much." [Rueful. Very rueful.]

Actually, I do have to admit that one of the brightest moments in my surgical career occurred after a surgical resident spent five minutes explaining to me how to do what he evidently viewed as a very complex suture maneuver ("Now, pass the left hand over and through, maintaining proper tension all the time on both strands . . ."), and I suddenly realized that he was just talking about a regular old blanket stitch, and was able to dazzle him with the rapidity with which I picked up the idea and laid down an even row of them. I didn't want to say anything about having practiced on blankets. Surgery is supposed to be super-macho, of course, so they have tried to elevate sewing into the realm of aerospace engineering, and if a woman seems to pick it up quickly, they mutter to each other that of course women have such small fingers. Many male surgeons want to be proud of their sewing in the manner of an expert laying complex circuitry, not a seamstress showing off her quilt, so why make trouble? You keep your mouth shut and you patch your quilt, and then you let them bang you on the back and tell you, "Strong work."

"Staples, are you serious? You put staples in skin?"

"There's this great little machine you use." [Matter-of-fact.] "And then there's this other machine, like a staple remover, that you use to take them out."

And your listener assumes that you are using the homely metaphor of the stapler to describe some fabulously precise medical process, whereas what you are talking about is a stapler and a staple remover. In fact, one surprise of surgery is that a great deal of it is much more crude than you imagined. This is not necessarily criticism; it's just that people tend to imagine mystic processes, remarkable instruments, and certainly there are enough of those in the surgical world, from fiber-optic arthroscopes which let you see inside the knee to lasers for microsurgery. Still, a lot of surgery is basically cut-the-patient-open-and-take-out-the-diseased-organ. The verb the surgeons themselves use is "whomp"—"We'll get him on the table and whomp out his gall bladder, and while we're in there, maybe we'll whomp out a piece of his bowel. . . ." This is not meant to belittle surgical abilities; all this whomping requires a great deal of judgment and manual dexterity, and there is always the possibility of disasters to be coped with. It's just that the actual operation itself is no mystic process: you whomp it out and then it's gone.

And that of course is the appeal of surgery, and also the "fun" of it, in medical student terms. There is something deeply satisfying about being part of the team that has just whomped out someone's tumor, or the enormous deposit that was obstructing a key artery, or the diseased appendix. You have actually cut out the disease. And even as a lowly retractor-holder, you get a little thrill of accomplishment, thinking of the patient waking up, free of that burden. This is an oversimplification, of course; there are many operations that cannot be considered at all in such simplistic terms. But still, it is much much truer in surgery than in internal medicine, where you almost never do a single definitive thing and actually "cure" a patient's disease.

"But aren't you scared? I mean, what if you make a mistake?"

"Well, you try to be careful." [Tough-minded.] "Still, mistakes are how you learn."

The other traditional medical student job in the OR is to cut sutures. The surgeon ties sutures, tying off blood vessels, repairing incisions in skin or muscle, and after each suture, there are the two long ends of thread. And then the medical student, holding the fancy surgical scissor in the approved way (don't imagine for a minute that you are doing anything the least little bit like a tailor trimming stitches), leans over and cuts off those ends, leaving just the right minute bits protruding from the knot. But, as surgical tradition would have it, there is no such thing as just the right minute bit. "No medical student has ever cut a suture perfectly," they said to me my first day. "They're either too long or too short." And I did not break this great tradition; all through surgery, I cut my sutures too long or too short, and considered myself lucky if I hadn't just spaced out during the operation, holding on to my retractor, to leave the surgeons calling in my direction, "Cut. Cut. Cut!"

Another favorite medical student error is to contaminate the sterile surgical field. Your first day in surgery you learn the drill, the hand-washing and the sterile gown-and-gloving; you learn not to put your hands below your waist, since waist-high and above is considered sterile; you learn not to touch someone's unsterile back with your sterile front; and you learn the complex geography of the OR, where there are in fact two parallel populations, the sterile or scrubbed, and the unsterile or unscrubbed. And then at some point you violate the inviolable, you touch a clean instrument to an unsterile towel, or you brush your unscrubbed hand against some sterile surgeon's arm, and then you've really gone and done it. I suppose it's part of your initiation into surgery, that particular disaster.

"What are the surgeons like? Do they really have temper tantrums?"

"Well, some of them are pretty odd, I have to admit." [Loyally, admiringly.] "Still, they do a really good job, they know what they're doing."

I have to admit, my time in surgery made me feel that I was finally discovering what it was like to be part of a high school boys' athletic team. The locker-room camaraderie. The insults to each other's masculinity (including mine). The poopoo jokes. The nicknames. The boasting about the highly improbable conquests, medical, sexual, or other. The highest praise: "Awesome!"

And then there are the jokes, which aren't quite jokes. Medical students have a reputation for a certain sort of sick humor, part defense, part bravado, and part genuine hilarity at the expense of the bizarre situations in which they find themselves. And surgeons have their jokes as well, their own sense of what is serious and what is funny. I think of Dr. Robinson, a resident who informed us that he was working out the details of an operation which would make him famous, to be called the "modified Robinson procedure." It would involve the removal of all nonessential organs at birth, to save surgery later on in life. (This was in the spirit of the surgeon who says, well, his appendix isn't inflamed after all, but as long as we've got him opened up, we might as well take out the appendix, and save him having it out later on.) The modified Robinson was a joke, but only marginally so.

The thing is, surgeons basically think that surgery is fun, just as medical students do. Ask them why they went into it, that's what they'll say, as often as not. The bigger the operation, the more awesome the whomp, the more fun it is. And though they can be absolute dictators in the operating room, and I have indeed seen a tantrum or two, what really stands out is the remarkable coolness under pressure. These are people who really come most fully alive in those odd scrubbed hours in the swimming-pool light of the OR, among the tiles and fluorescence and the reverberating voices.

I never wanted to be a surgeon. Still, medical school has had me doing any number of things I never wanted to do, and surgery, by comparison to most, was sort of fun. By the end of my time in surgery I was actually itching to do some cutting, and when they let me take out an infected cyst all by myself, I carried on about my "case" as if I had done complex work under bright lights for hours to save someone's life, or eyesight, or leg . . . and the rest of my team patted me on the back and said, sure enough, "Awesome!"

* * *

"How many surgeons does it take to change a light bulb?"

"Why don't you just have us remove the socket? You aren't using it, and it'll only cause you trouble in the future."

Emergency Room

Two years of medical school, and you don't know what to do for someone with back pain. Well, why should you? What did they ever teach you about back pain? So you stand there in the emergency room, looking sympathetic, while this clean-cut young man explains that he gets this every so often, and there's a certain painkiller that helps, and he usually gets it from his university health service (he goes to an Ivy League college in a different state), but he's here now on vacation, and the back pain is going to ruin it.

Two years of medical school, and you have no idea what to do for someone with back pain. X rays? Radioactive bone scans? Surgery? Tell him to sleep on the floor, as your mother did when she had backaches? Heating pads? Exercise? Don't exercise? You push away some knee-jerk medical student thoughts like, rule out pancreatic cancer, rule out aortic aneurysm.

You poke around at his spine for a while, feel his back muscles, ask, does this hurt? how about this? how about when I do this? You ask him to bend over in a couple of directions, and then you make some official-looking notes on your clipboard ("21-yr-old m back hurts wants pain meds") and go off in search of advice.

The emergency room is fairly calm, and you find the doctor in charge, the attending, and tell him your story. When you're through, the attending asks, "Are

you convinced? Sounds a little like he might be looking for narcotics, doesn't it, with this story about being
from out of state, and wanting this specific drug? I'll
talk to him when I get a chance—meanwhile, go have
a look at the patient in Bed Three. Textbook case."

The patient in Bed 3 is a woman in her forties who
has belly pain. You ask her a set of questions about
where it is and what brought it on and what makes it
better or worse and has she ever had anything like it
before. While you're poking at her abdomen, an intern arrives; the patient is being admitted to the hospital, and the intern has come to get her story and
examine her. Politely, you get out of the way.

"So what do you think she has?" asks the attending.

"Gall bladder," you say.

"I think you're right. What are the six *F*s of gall
bladder disease?"

That you know; it's a perfect question for a medical
student. "Fair, fat, female, fertile, fortyish . . ." Wait
a minute, that's only five.

"Flatulent," says the attending, and you file it away
for future reference. "What are the other things you
worry about?" You begin to reel off a list: appendicitis, ectopic pregnancy, pancreatitis, and the attending
stops you to say, "Look over there in the pediatric
room. I think a lac just came in."

A lac is a laceration, a cut, and everyone knows
medical students like lacs; you get to stitch them up,
and you feel like a real doctor. Since no one else is
very much interested in lacs, the medical student on
duty usually gets them. So you go over to the pediatric
room and find a distraught mother and a three-year-
old girl with a gash on her arm.

At your approach, the child, who has been perfectly
calm, begins to shriek; probably she associates your
white coat with getting shots. "Now, how did this
happen?" you ask cheerfully.

The mother, hugging the child, is telling you how it happened. You try to examine the wound and, though the child is still screaming her head off, also listen carefully to the story; you know that when you go out to tell the attending about this he'll ask you, as he always does, if you're satisfied there's no child abuse involved. So you press the mother a little for details, and observe how she holds and comforts her daughter, and decide, for better or worse, that you aren't concerned about child abuse here. "Well, that's going to need a couple of stitches, I think," you tell the mother. The child has no intention of cooperating. When a lot of strangers in white coats begin to talk to her soothingly about giving her one little needle so she won't feel anything at all, and then they'll fix her arm as good as new, she very sensibly refuses to have anything to do with it. She ends up in a papoose board, large Velcro straps holding her as motionless as possible, as you inject her arm with a local anesthetic and carefully suture up the laceration. You do feel like a doctor as you do this, even though you know the reason you can set sutures so neatly and evenly has nothing to do with medical school; you've always been good at sewing and embroidery.

The child is released from the papoose board, the mother thanks you profusely, and, feeling like a doctor, you head off to see what's become of your Ivy League back-pain patient. The attending has talked to him and is very dubious. The young man wants a specific painkiller, one that's a common drug of abuse; he wants a large supply of it; there's no one doctor you can call to check with; and lower back pain is, of course, one of those things you can't verify with any medical test.

"So, what do you want to do?" asks the attending.

Well, you don't really consider it your job to act as some kind of police officer, regulating the flow of drugs—that isn't why you went into medicine. And suppose the guy really is in pain? Timidly, you recommend giving him a small supply of painkillers and suggesting that if he wants more he should get in touch with his doctor back home. Fine, says the attending, and sends you off to explain this to the patient. The patient, needless to say, isn't pleased, though you explain to him over and over that this is strictly routine. "This is a big-city emergency room," you keep saying. "We can't give out prescriptions for large amounts of narcotics."

So you go back to the attending, who tells you to write out the prescription. Well. Two years of medical school and you don't know how to write a prescription. You stare down at the little pad, wondering what the dose is, how to specify the number of pills. The attending looks up, notices your confusion, and dictates the prescription. You write it down, the attending signs it, and you carry it to the patient, who snatches it, furious, and departs. This doesn't make you feel particularly like a doctor.

For the medical student, life is full of opportunities to show off your ignorance. On the wards, they ask you about complications, obscure diagnoses. In the emergency room, you're brought up against the realization that you have no idea how to treat a nosebleed, a cat bite, a fishhook through the finger. What do you do first for a girl who has been hit in the eye with a hockey stick? What do you do for someone who calmly tells you that he took a bunch of pills he found in the medicine chest, that he has no idea what they were, that he didn't really want to kill himself, and that he feels fine? You have to make quick nonmedical judgments about people: you have to decide after a few minutes' acquaintance whether you suspect child abuse, whether you want to give the prescription for narcotics.

Nonetheless, it's exciting to work in the emergency room, to be the first person the patient sees, to be involved in all the most basic decisions: what do you think is wrong with this person? what should we do first? is this a hospital admission? do you believe this story? On the wards, most of the patients come to you already diagnosed by their own doctors or in the emergency room; there are often still questions to answer, but there's a sense that the stories have already been sorted out a little. In the emergency room, the patients come in off the street, and you do the sorting. In one bed is an elderly man who has broken his hip, in the next a high school student who got hit on the elbow with a baseball and wants a note excusing him from gym for at least a month. Across the room is a woman who has chest pain and may have had a heart attack, and next to her is a man with Alzheimer's disease whose behavior has changed abruptly. Has he had a stroke?

The rhythm of the emergency room is very different from that of the wards; it's a rhythm of tiny crises and big emergencies. The telephone rings to announce that the rescue squad is bringing in a woman found on the street, not breathing, get ready to resuscitate. Meanwhile, you go see someone with a sore throat.

There's plenty of human drama in an emergency room, as anywhere in a hospital, and there are all sorts of peculiar, unanswerable questions: why does someone who has lived with a vague pain in his ankle for over a week suddenly decide to come to the emergency room at 3:00 A.M. on a miserable, cold, rainy night?

Everyone who comes to an emergency room comes thinking, this is an emergency. My pain, my injury, my worry—this is something that merits a trip to the hospital, hours out of my day, a long wait, filling out a bunch of forms, paying the bill. And the patient often finds out that by the standards of the emergency room it isn't such a big deal. Have a seat, says the triage nurse, deciding that this one isn't about to drop dead. The real life-and-death emergencies tend to arrive by ambulance, carried in through a different entrance, while the people in the waiting room sit and wait. In a way, what you see here is one of the essential dilemmas of practicing medicine, concentrated by the particular pressures of the emergency room. The patient comes in hurting, thinking, my pain is an emergency. The doctor weighs and measures the pain, and concludes that the pain in Bed 5 is a minor annoyance compared to the pain in Bed 3, and yet the patient in Bed 5 is entitled to care, reassurance, explanations— not just the news that someone in Bed 3 is worse off.

You do what you can, giving patients more or less time, depending on how busy things are. Frequently comfort is all you have to offer; sometimes you're able to help, but often you're not sure whether you really know what it is you're helping.

A standard medical joke is the one about the duck hunt; it exists in several versions, depending on which specialty is doing the telling, which specialty it's aimed at. The emergency medicine version goes like this: Four doctors go duck hunting, a surgeon, an internist, a radiologist, and an emergency room doctor. The surgeon looks up at the sky. "There's a goddam duck!" he says, and shoots. The duck falls to the ground, dead. Then the internist looks up. "Duck," he says. "Rule out pigeon, rule out eagle. . . ." The duck flies away. The radiologist looks up. "I think it's a duck, but to be sure, we need a chest film," he says, and the duck flies away. Then the emergency room doctor suddenly blasts away with his gun. "I got it, I got it!" he yells. "What the hell was it?"

Babytalk

My first clinic patient is one of the older ones. Seventeen, and six months pregnant. Doesn't look pregnant at all. I measure her uterus with a tape measure, record my results on her clinic sheet.

"Your baby's growing well," I tell her. "But you might try to gain a little bit more weight for next month."

"I don't want to get fat," she says.

"But you need to gain weight when you're pregnant. Your baby needs you to. Are you living with your parents?"

"Are you kidding me?" she says, with total scorn. Puts her boots on, adjusts the elaborate web of chains and charms around her neck. Looks at me as if to say, your clothes are dumb, your earrings are cornball, get off my case. Or at least, that's what I imagine. I was seventeen myself once, and pretty damn scornful, and I have trouble finding a tone of voice that I think will work.

The next patient is docile. Of course, she's only fifteen, and she's here with her mother. The girl is seven months pregnant. As she lies on the table, I find the fetal heartbeat with the little ultrasound machine, and smile. "Hear that?" I ask, and my patient smiles, then looks at her mother.

"Good and strong," the mother says.

"Do you have any questions?" I ask.

"Am I going to be allowed to be with her when she goes into labor?" asks the mother. "I know they let the father stay, but he's not going to be there. Even if he was, he wouldn't be any use."

"Oh, Mom," says the daughter, gently, still smiling.

"Sure, you'll be able to stay," I say. "Are you going to go to the classes together?"

"Yes, we are," the mother says, and she puts an arm around her spherical daughter, who has just struggled off the examining table. In the little room there's a palpable and pleasant sense of maternal affection, of a strong mother protecting a rather innocent child. But the obviously maternal silhouette of the child makes it all rather convoluted, and though these two listen carefully to all my good advice, I'm not sorry to see them go.

These patients are ten, eleven, twelve years younger than I am. They make me feel deeply naive, because they consistently shock me. I mean, reading about teenage pregnancy in the newspaper is just not the same as spending a morning in a prepartum clinic like this one, taking care of what seem to be the entire sophomore and junior classes of a nearby high school. As I go out into the waiting room to call my next patient, I overhear the following exchange:

"Did you hear Laurie had her baby?"

"Really? What'd she have?"

"A boy."

"A boy, that's great. She used to sit next to me in study hall."

And mind you, the sophomores and juniors at least look old enough to be in high school. There are occasional twelve- and thirteen-year-olds as well. My next patient, who's sixteen, is five months pregnant with her *second* child.

"How does your son feel about the new baby coming?" I ask, idiotically.

"He didn't tell me. He's only one year old, you know."

"Well," I say, cheerfully, "have you given any thought to what birth control you're going to use after the baby's born?"

"I'm going on the Pill."

"Oh, that's fine. That's a good, reliable method."

"Yeah. I was using it before, after my other baby was born."

"So how did you get pregnant again?"

She shrugs. I know the possible answers—forgot to take it, meant to take it, et cetera, et cetera.

"How do your parents feel about the new baby?"

"Oh, my mother's okay. My father, first he wanted me to have an abortion. But he's coming around."

"Why don't they have abortions?" I ask the obstetrician/gynecologist who's supervising me. "When I was in high school, girls who got pregnant had abortions."

"When I was in high school most people didn't have sex at all, and I'm only ten years older than you are."

"Well, lots of people in my high school had sex, but they didn't have babies."

That's the way it is in the college-bound suburbs, I suppose. As for why these patients don't have abortions, you've probably heard (or read) all the reasons. A baby will solve my life, a baby will love me, a baby will make me a grownup. These girls seem eager to abandon the supposedly privileged state of adolescence, which never turns out to be anything like the way it is in the movies, and they believe that motherhood will better live up to its Hallmark-card reputation.

"It didn't get so much attention when people thought it was mostly black teenagers having babies," says the doctor. "Now that they've realized it's all kinds of teenagers, suddenly it's a media event."

*   *   *

One morning in the hospital things were quiet up on Labor and Delivery, and I was sitting with an obstetrician and three nurses, watching a TV talk show. The guests were two teenage mothers, a doctor, and a woman from an antiabortion group. No one actually talked to anyone else; the hostess would ask one of them a question, the guest would make a flat statement, and no one would respond. The hostess was trying to get them to commit themselves: *Should contraceptives be given out in schools?* One of the mothers said she hadn't known anything at all about contraceptives before she got pregnant. The doctor said you shouldn't ever give out contraceptives without counseling. The woman from the antiabortion group said, no, we must not give out contraceptives, that's not the answer. So what is the answer, asked the moderator. The woman smiled beatifically. We have failed our children, she said, we have failed them on many levels, we have failed to provide them with love and with moral leadership, and that's where the answer lies.

In the hospital TV room the obstetrician called out: "Yes, but in the meantime could you give out some contraceptives?"

Debbie is sixteen, and in labor with her first baby. The contractions are regular, every ten minutes or so, and they're starting to get painful. She has just arrived at the hospital, and one of the nurses has finished setting her up in a labor room.

I introduce myself: Hi, I'm a medical student, I'll be staying with you while you're in labor, if that's okay with you.

"I don't care who you are," Debbie says, "just so you give me something to knock me out." She hasn't been to any childbirth preparation classes, has seen a doctor twice during her pregnancy. One of her friends from high school just had a baby, and warned her that "natural childbirth" hurts like hell, and the doctors always try to con you into it. Her mother, who should be arriving soon, has told her that there's a drug you can give a woman in labor that puts her right to sleep, and then she wakes up after the baby is born.

"Um, we don't give that drug anymore," I say, as gently as I can. "It isn't really safe for you or for your baby. But we can give you medicines to make it all easier if you need them."

Debbie is completely unwilling to believe me. She has been counting on sleeping through labor and delivery, reminding herself that as soon as the pain starts, she will be put out. She's positive that it's punitive, my denying her this drug her mother told her she could have. She's terrified; all her emotional props for facing labor have just been destroyed. She begins to scream at me, curse at me. And for a split second I imagine that I can hear something else in her attack, the furious resentment of a sixteen-year-old who, without ever consciously choosing, has decided her life. Resenting me? Why should she resent me? She doesn't know that I'm thinking, automatically, *when I was your age, I would never have had a baby*. No, she's just angry with me because of the drug I won't give her.

Debbie's mother arrives, along with Debbie's boyfriend, who to my eye looks about fourteen. And terrified. But his presence, and her mother's, calm Debbie a little. The doctor comes by and gives her some Demerol. Her mother assures her that she doesn't need to be put to sleep, the drugs will keep her from feeling pain. Not exactly true, but I don't correct her.

Debbie's labor moves along fairly quickly. She's actually quite lucky: the nurses have lots of stories of teenagers in labor for days. Her boyfriend becomes suddenly faint when the bag of amniotic fluid breaks with an impressive gush; a nurse helps him to sit down, put his head between his legs. Debbie is concerned for him, and somehow his trouble seems to help her stay in control. She really manages very well for someone who had no idea what to expect from labor.

After the baby is born, though, Debbie doesn't want to hold her. "You take her, Mom," she says. "You know what to do."

"She's your baby, you know," the nurse says. "You have to learn to take care of her."

"Later, okay, Mom?" Debbie says, with perfect adolescent intonation.

Invasions

Morning rounds in the hospital. We charge along, the resident leading the way, the interns following, the two medical students last, pushing the cart that holds the patients' charts. The resident pulls up in front of a patient's door, the interns stop as well, and we almost run them over with the chart cart. It's time to present the patient, a man who came into the hospital late last night. I did the workup—interviewed him, got his medical history, examined him, wrote a six-page note in his chart, and (at least in theory) spent a little while in the hospital library, reading up on his problems.

"You have sixty seconds, go!" says the resident, looking at his watch. I am of course thinking rebelliously that the interns take as long as they like with their presentations, that the resident himself is long-winded and full of pointless anecdotes—but at the same time I am swinging into my presentation, talking as fast as I can to remind my listeners that no time is being wasted, using the standard hospital turns of phrase. "Mr. Z. is a seventy-eight-year-old white male who presents with dysuria and intermittent hematuria of one week's duration." In other words, for the past week Mr. Z. has experienced pain with urination, and has occasionally passed blood. I rocket on, thinking only about getting through the presentation without being told off for taking too long, without being repri-manded for including nonessential items—or for leav-

ing out crucial bits of data. Of course, fair is fair, my
judgment about what is critical and what is not is very
faulty. Should I include in this very short presentation
(known as a "bullet") that Mr. Z. had gonorrhea five
years ago? Well, yes, I decide, and include it in my
sentence, beginning, "Pertinent past medical history
includes . . ." I don't even have a second to remember
how Mr. Z. told me about his gonorrhea, how he
made me repeat the question three times last night,
my supposedly casual question dropped in between
"Have you ever been exposed to tuberculosis?" and
"Have you traveled out of the country recently?"

"Five years ago?" The resident interrupts me. "When
he was seventy-three? Well, good for him!"

Feeling almost guilty, I think of last night, of how
Mr. Z.'s voice dropped to a whisper when he told me
about the gonorrhea, how he then went on, as if he
felt he had no choice, to explain that he had gone to a
convention and "been with a hooker—excuse me, miss,
no offense," and how he had then infected his wife,
and so on. I am fairly used to this by now, the impulse
people sometimes have to confide everything to the
person examining them as they enter the hospital. I
don't know whether they are frightened by suggestions
of disease and mortality, or just accepting me as a
medical professional and using me as a comfortable
repository for secrets. I have had people tell me about
their childhoods and the deaths of their relatives, about
their jobs, about things I have needed to ask about
and things that have no conceivable bearing on anything that concerns me.

In we charge to examine Mr. Z. The resident introduces himself and the other members of the team, and
then he and the interns listen to Mr. Z.'s chest, feel
his stomach. As they pull up Mr. Z.'s gown to examine his genitals, the resident says heartily, "Well now,
I understand you had a little trouble with VD not so

long ago." And immediately I feel like a traitor; I am sure that Mr. Z. is looking at me reproachfully. I have betrayed the secret he was so hesitant to trust me with.

I am aware that my scruples are ridiculous. It is possibly relevant that Mr. Z. had gonorrhea; it is certainly relevant to know how he was treated, whether he might have been reinfected. And in fact, when I make myself meet his eyes, he does not look nearly as distressed at being examined by three people and asked this question in a loud booming voice as he seemed last night with my would-be-tactful inquiries.

In fact, Mr. Z. is getting used to being in the hospital. And in the hospital, as a patient, you have no privacy. The privacy of your body is of necessity violated constantly by doctors and nurses (and the occasional medical student), and details about your physical condition are discussed by the people taking care of you. And your body is made to give up its secrets with a variety of sophisticated techniques, from blood tests to X rays to biopsies—the whole point is to deny your body the privacy that pathological processes need in order to do their damage. Everything must be brought to light, exposed, analyzed, and noted in the chart. And all this is essential for medical care, and even the most modest patients are usually able to come to terms with it, exempting medical personnel from all the most basic rules of privacy and distance.

So much for the details of the patient's physical condition. But the same thing can happen to details of the patient's life. For the remainder of Mr. Z.'s hospital stay, my resident was fond of saying to other doctors, "Got a guy on our service, seventy-eight, got gonorrhea when he was seventy-three, from a showgirl. Pretty good, huh?" He wouldn't ever have said such a thing to Mr. Z.'s relatives, of course, or to any nondoctor. But when it came to his fellow doctors, he saw nothing wrong with it.

I remember another night, 4:00 A.M. in the hospital and I had finally gone to sleep after working-up a young woman with a bad case of stomach cramps and diarrhea. Gratefully, I climbed into the top bunk in the on-call room, leaving the bottom bunk for the intern, who might never get to bed, and who, if she did, would have to be ready to leap up at a moment's notice if there was an emergency. Me, I hoped that, emergency or not, I would be overlooked in the top bunk and allowed to sleep out the next two hours and fifty-five minutes in peace (I reserved five minutes to pull myself together before rounds). I lay down and closed my eyes, and something occurred to me. With typical medical student compulsiveness, I had done what is called a "mega-workup" on this patient, I had asked her every possible question about her history and conscientiously written down all her answers. And suddenly I realized that I had written in her chart careful details of all her drug use, cocaine, amphetamines, hallucinogens, all the things she had said she had once used but didn't anymore. She was about my age and had talked to me easily, cheerfully, once her pain was relatively under control, telling me she used to be really into this and that, but now she didn't even drink. And I had written all the details in her chart. I couldn't go to sleep, thinking about those sentences. There was no reason for them. There was no reason everyone had to know all this. There was no reason it had to be written in her official chart, available for legal subpoena. It was four in the morning and I was weary and by no means clear-headed; I began to fantasize one scenario after another in which my careless remarks in this woman's record cost her a job, got her thrown into jail, discredited her forever. And as I dragged myself out of the top bunk and out to the nurses' station to find her chart and cross out the offending sentences with such heavy black lines that they could never be read, I was conscious of an agreeable sense of self-sacrifice—here I was, smudging my immaculate mega-writeup to protect my patient. On rounds, I would just say, "Some past drug use," if it seemed relevant.

Medical records are tricky items legally. Medical students are always being reminded to be discreet about what they write—the patient can demand to see the record, the records can be subpoenaed in a trial. Do not make jokes. If you think a serious mistake has been made, do not write that in the record—that is not for you to judge, and you will be providing ammunition for anyone trying to use the record against the hospital. And gradually, in fact, you learn a set of evasions and euphemisms with which doctors comment in charts on differences of opinion, misdiagnoses, and even errors. "Unfortunate complication of usually benign procedure." That kind of thing. The chart is a potential source of damage; damage to the patient, as I was afraid of doing, or damage to the hospital and the doctor.

Medical students and doctors have a reputation for crude humor; some is merely off-color, which comes naturally to people who deal all day with sick bodies. Other jokes can be more disturbing; I remember a patient whose cancer had destroyed her vocal chords so she could no longer talk. In taking her history from her daughter we happened to find out that she had once been a professional musician, singing and playing the piano in supper clubs. For the rest of her stay in the hospital, the resident always introduced her case, when discussing it with other doctors, by saying, "Do you know Mrs. Q.? She used to sing and play the piano—now she just plays the piano."

As you learn to become a doctor, there is a frequent

sense of surprise, a feeling that you are not entitled to
the kind of intrusion you are allowed into patients'
lives. Without arguing, they permit you to examine
them; it is impossible to imagine, when you do your
very first physical exam, that someday you will walk in
calmly and tell a man your grandfather's age to un-
dress, and then examine him without thinking about it
twice. You get used to it all, but every so often you
find yourself marveling at the access you are allowed,
at the way you are learning from the bodies, the
stories, the lives and deaths of perfect strangers. They
give up their privacy in exchange for some hope—
sometimes strong, sometimes faint—of the alleviation
of pain, the curing of disease. And gradually, with
medical training, that feeling of amazement, that feeling that you are not entitled, scars over. You begin to
identify more thoroughly with the medical profession—
of course you are entitled to see everything and know
everything; you're a doctor, aren't you? And as you
accept this as your right, you move farther from your
patients, even as you penetrate more meticulously and
more confidently into their lives.

007s

Let's talk about something you probably don't want to hear about. The bad medical students, the ones who aren't any good at what they do. The ones who don't know what they're talking about. As they say in the hospital, the OO7s—licensed to kill. (Well, no, not exactly—that's what they say about medical students who turn a simple IV into a major trauma; it usually takes a full-fledged 007 *doctor* to kill you.)

There always has to be a spectrum, of course. Take a hundred fifty or so bright kids, all good on tests, all good in their college science courses, all with a few interesting experiences in or around research, all with the proverbial volunteer work in a hospital emergency room (". . . really helped me to understand what medicine is all about, and confirmed me in my decision to devote my life to this challenging and rewarding profession . . ."). Put them together in a medical school class, tell them to relax, they're all going to be doctors, remind them that everything is pass/fail from now on (P = MD, the upperclassmen explain), and what do you have? Well, a spectrum, of course. Some are better than others, and everyone is keenly aware of that. And for the first couple of years of medical school this raises those familiar questions, who does well on tests, who performs brilliantly in discussion section. But then it's time to move on into the hospitals, and you begin to consider, and reconsider. What will it mean to be one of the ones who is not so good at it? Will it mean killing patients whom other people could have saved? What will the spectrum mean when we are actually "on the wards"?

What they tell you, of course, is that the spectrum is from good to better to best—that was the point of all those tests and that prolonged admissions process. You're all going to be just fine, and some of you will be superb (and will come do your residencies in our very own hospitals) and the rest of you will be merely excellent. And this, of course, is nonsense.

So there you are, sick in bed, and they walk in. The resident and the medical student and the nurse, carrying various pieces of equipment.

"Now we're going to do that procedure I was telling you about, the spinal tap," the resident says cheerfully.

The nurse helps bend you into fetal position.

"Remember, position is everything when you're doing a spinal tap," says the resident.

You realize that it is the medical student who is to do the procedure. "Have you ever done this before?" you ask, trying to keep your voice light.

The resident answers for the student, who is preoccupied with trying to get the kit open. "Of course he has!" the resident says heartily. "He's one of our real experts."

Behind your back, where you can't see, the resident mouths to the nurse, "He's done lots of them—and he's missed every goddam one."

As a medical student starting out on the wards, the first fears usually concern procedures, manual skills. I'll never be able to start an IV line. I tried five times and finally I went and told the intern that it was a really difficult patient, and he got it in on the first try and said the patient had perfect veins. I never want to start an IV again. I'll never be able to draw blood gases. I repeated that spinal tap three times and I didn't get any spinal fluid.

Some people are simply talented at all these procedures, and some people are terrible. And no question, medical students who are terrible at drawing blood put their patients through a lot of unnecessary torture, sticking them again and again, muttering to them, "You have very small veins," or "They've already drawn so much blood from you, they've spoiled all your veins."

This is the medical student's terror, and probably the patient's most likely terror (after all, if you can get a goofus medical student fumbling over you, why not a goofus surgeon in the operating room?). But in fact, sooner or later all medical students learn to do procedures—roughly or gently, first try or fourth. Clumsiness never stopped anyone, in the end.

So you're still bent with your knees to your chest, and the medical student is making yet another attempt at the spinal tap—his fourth, or is it his fifth? The resident is leaning against the wall, casually saying, "Be careful with your left hand, you're about to contaminate the field," and "Now slow down and find your landmarks, don't just stick blindly."

And you are lying there, sick and feverish, wondering why you are allowing this obvious goofus (you mistrusted him from the moment you saw him) to stick needles into your spine. (But if you stop him, will you antagonize the resident?)

The resident looks a little impatient. The medical student is behind your back so you can't see him, but the resident's impatience may be making him impatient too—he drops a piece of equipment. With elaborate calm, the resident says to the nurse, "Could you get us another needle, please?" She starts out the door and the resident calls, "Actually, you'd better get four or five."

If you had any sympathy to spare, you might actually feel sorry for the wretched student. But you're too busy feeling sorry for yourself, trying not to anger the resident, and at the same time reproaching yourself as a hopeless coward (the word *spineless* occurs to you but you repress the thought). Over and over you tell yourself that it must be okay, this student is a carefully selected individual studying at a highly prestigious institution.

"So then," the resident says, conversationally, "tell me once more what happens to the spinal-fluid protein level in bacterial meningitis."

"It goes down," says the medical student, in the tones of one guessing on a fifty-fifty proposition.

"Nope, it's elevated. How about the glucose level?"

"That's up too," says your tormentor, finding a new place to stick a needle in your back.

"Nope, glucose down, protein up. Watch it now, find your landmarks, don't stick blindly."

What does it mean to be a lousy medical student? Different things to different people. To the interns and the residents, it can mean a student who is not skilled enough to be sent off to start IVs, or a student who acts grumpy and unwilling if woken up at night. (*Bad attitude.* That's how it's phrased in the evaluations charting medical students' progress through the hospital.) To the attending physician, it is more likely to mean a student who is unable to answer obscure questions when put on the spot suddenly in front of a group. (*Doesn't perform well under pressure.*)

Medical students are often afraid of being found out in abysmal ignorance; all the hasty studying, the memorizing and forgetting, of the first two years of medical school seem to lie in wait to trip them up. And it's true, students do have to learn a certain amount, and it's possible to get in trouble if your answers are always wrong. But roundsmanship is a game, and eventually pretty much everyone learns the rules. Comparative ignorance never stopped anyone, in the end.

The resident takes over and does the tap, then leaves the room, telling the medical student to answer any questions you may have. You stretch out your legs and lie still, happy that it's over, as the nurse cleans up your back.

"So gee," says the medical student, "this can give you brain damage, you know?"

There are comparatively few people who cannot eventually master the technical side of medicine, and cannot ultimately learn enough to struggle along to a reasonable diagnosis. But what about the students who are simply incompetent at dealing with people? That, after all, is a much harder skill to teach. In medical school my classmates used to joke about taking up a collection for a scholarship fund to pay all the future training expenses of a certain student, as long as he went into research and promised never to talk to or touch a patient.

And in fact, though he probably knows he is terrible at procedures, though repeated humiliations on rounds may tell him that his "fund of knowledge is weak" (as the evaluations put it), though eventually when he is further along in his training, people will notice if his patients die unnecessarily, there is really no way for anyone to notice that he is rotten at what is called, in our curriculum, The Doctor-Patient Relationship. He does a lousy job of telling people what's wrong with them. A terrible job of telling them they're dying. Totally insensitive with the families of patients. Bedside manner that makes your skin crawl.

His colleagues may know. The nurses will know. But in fact, this kind of incompetence, impossible to quantify, is rarely grounds for any kind of formal correction.

A joke about the bad medical student, and how he comes out on top: The notoriously bad medical student is being grilled on rounds. The attending is describing a patient who showed up in the emergency room with lower back pain. The story involves a complex history, a multitude of confusing symptoms. The attending asks, "So, what's your diagnosis?"

"Ruptured aortic aneurysm," says the student without hesitation, naming a rare and catastrophic condition in which the aorta can tear, a condition requiring immediate surgery.

"That's right!" says the attending, amazed. "How on earth did you figure it out?"

"What else gives you lower back pain?" asks the student, in honest perplexity.

Enough to Make You Sick

Late at night in the hospital, I had, I will admit, any number of odd and less than noble thoughts. I am talking about the medical student (me), in the hospital on a thirty-hour shift, prevented from sleeping by the uncontrollable changes in condition of the sick, or sometimes by my own need to stay awake and learn something before morning rounds. I am talking about those dark hours of the soul when one is reduced to scrounging yet again in one's pocket for enough change to coax yet another candy bar out of the vending machine in the cafeteria for a few seconds of sugar rush. Those hours when the human spirit is at its lowest ebb, and the medical student stares out the window into the night and tries to think of some friend in California—it's 4:00 A.M. here, so it'll be only 1:00 A.M. there—who'll still be awake and willing to talk. But will she accept a collect call?

Yes, many thoughts flicker across the mind. Professions-I-could-have-gone-into, for example, each with bountiful professional rewards, the luxury of daytime working hours, no blood on your clothes . . . Or how about just the more general for-this-I-am-going-eighty-thousand-dollars-into-debt? train of thought. Or the all-my-friends-who-don't-go-to-medical-school-are-in-warm-beds-asleep-and-probably-with-each-other-and-I-hate-them-all chain of reasoning.

But every now and then I went farther than this.

Feeling sorry for myself was all well and good, and nursed me along until the next candy-bar attack, but when things really got bad, I would find myself standing by some patient's bed, envying that patient with all my strength. Yes, there I would stand, staring at some poor sick person, probably in pain, certainly desperate to be well again, and I would think, well, I would be willing to take on a small case of that disease, if it would mean . . . if it would mean what? Well, most immediately, the right to get into the bed and close my eyes, with no responsibility for anyone who might suddenly develop a fever or begin breathing too fast, with no need to memorize all the possible causes of neck pain by 8:00 A.M.

But it would mean more than that, though it was the thought of putting my head down on the pillow that really made me salivate. It would also mean having people attentive to my needs, nurses and doctors coming by to see how I was doing. Tender loving care. Instead of candy bars, carefully balanced and scientifically engineered hospital meals; inedible, granted, but certainly good for me. Instead of constant summonses to wake up at night, solicitous nurses asking why I wasn't asleep, offering me medication to help me sleep more soundly. People would feel sorry for me. Instead of being an ignorant in-the-way medical student, to be corrected and reprimanded and at all costs prevented from committing serious medical malpractice, I would be a poor suffering martyr, the focus of attention for all the people who pick on medical students.

Oh, the shame of it. Standing there, a young healthy woman, with her life in front of her, envying the sick. Striking bargains with whatever powers might be listening: no, it wouldn't be worth it to have stomach cancer, but I wouldn't mind a little gall bladder disease. Well, maybe not a bacterial meningitis, but how about a mild pneumonia.

This was sick, in more ways than one. It reflected an extreme situation, as well as my own willingness to feel sorry for myself, and the concurrent strong desire to have others feeling sorry for me as well, to *deserve* their pity because of my miserable sick state, rather than because I was on my way to an MD.

However, more seriously, what is called the "sick role" may have its rewards for other people as well; less extreme circumstances than the hospital in the middle of the night may offer less extreme trade-offs and more subtle rewards. There are two angles from which I want to look at the potential pleasures of the sick role. First, what are the possible scenarios in which a patient may claim symptoms that do not in fact have an identifiable pathology to account for them? What is going on in the patient's mind? And second, what goes on in the doctor's mind when dealing with a patient who is, by the doctor's standards, not really sick?

First, the patient. There is a straightforward and essentially impossible question to be asked about a person who is describing symptoms that cannot be ascribed to any disease—is the patient actually feeling these symptoms, or are they being claimed in order to earn what is called in medicine "secondary gain," a term which can mean anything from compensation for being out of work to the love and sympathy of one's relatives.

Anyway, a woman brings her seven-year-old son into the emergency room one night. The child has been complaining of excruciating abdominal pain, so bad it makes him moan and groan and cry out. The mother is worried that it may be appendicitis, but also suspicious because she happens to know that there is a major spelling test scheduled for the next day, and her son is a terrible speller. Furthermore, his father has announced that if he brings home any more bad test papers, the child is going to have his computer taken away—and the boy cannot sleep without his computer beside him.

The emergency room doctor takes a very careful medical history from the child, looking into what the pain feels like, what makes it get worse, what makes it get better, is the patient hungry or thirsty, and so on and on. Then the boy is examined, and a couple of blood tests are sent. The doctor feels reasonably sure (not positive, just reasonably sure) that it is not appendicitis, nor any other medical condition she can treat. But that does not answer the question, is this boy pretending to have stomach pain so he can get out of going to school tomorrow and taking his test, or does the prospect of taking the test, facing his father, and losing his computer terrify him so thoroughly that his stomach is hurting him? These are two very different medical phenomena. The former, the production of symptoms for secondary gain, is called malingering. The latter, the transformation of a psychological difficulty into a physical symptom, is called somatization. Both patterns, in extreme cases, can be evidence of psychological disorders, but both patterns, to one degree or another, fit almost all of us.

It is in fact not at all difficult to imagine why the sick role should appeal to different people at different times. It is a way for a person to ask for love and attention without seeming to beg, it is a way to increase one's own importance within one's family group, it is a concrete way to express various dissatisfactions and longings which are making life unpleasant. And all this does not necessarily mean that the patient is toting it up on a mental balance sheet, making careful decisions about how sick to claim to be. Much of it may be completely unconscious. Much of it is learned—a child who learned, growing up, that the smallest disease deserved tremendous fuss may grow up to exag-

gerate his sensations in keeping with the seriousness of
the reaction he expects them to provoke. Dorothy
Parker wrote:

> *Weep, my love, till Heaven hears;*
> *Curse and moan and languish*
> *While I wash your wound with tears,*
> *Ease aloud your anguish.*
>
> *Bellow of the pit in Hell*
> *Where you're made to linger.*
> *There and there and well and well—*
> *Did he prick his finger!*

Literature is full of chronic invalids who are suspected,
if not actually accused, by their creators of being in it
a little for their own enjoyment. And yet society in
general continues to hold onto the myth that everything about being sick is highly unpleasant, so why on
earth would anyone who wasn't *really* sick . . . ? And
it is this assumption which robs the sick role of blame
and guilt, making it sometimes appear a haven to tired
medical students or to anyone at all.

But from the point of view of doctors, all this can
look very different. Never mind that someone may
feel very annoyed at spending an hour in a busy emergency room finding out that in fact the patient always
gets these pains right before a visit from her sister.
That annoyance is not justified; tension and anxiety
can spark all sorts of medical symptoms requiring treatment, from migraines to the local version of Montezu-
ma's revenge. More serious is the problem posed for
the doctor by someone with symptoms for which no
"explanation" can be found. That is, you've worked
this guy up from every possible angle. To be honest,
you thought he might have cancer, with the complex
of symptoms he described, but you've ruled out every

kind of cancer you can think of, as well as enough other things to fill a ten-pound textbook of medicine. You suspected all along that this was what you politely call a "supratentorial problem"—an anatomical way of saying it's all in his head. But when do you stop working him up? There is always another test you can do, another even more unlikely diagnosis to rule out (the medical student has just presented you with a list of five more; one of them is so rare that there are only four reported cases in all medical literature). *You might be missing something. What if he has a treatable disease and you just haven't found it?* These thoughts nag at you as you tell the medical student, okay, let's send some blood off to the one lab in the state that does that test—what have we got to lose? And it does occur to you, as the student goes in to draw the blood, that this really can't be much fun for the patient. (There actually is a psychiatric syndrome, Munchausen's syndrome, in which patients willingly if not eagerly incur invasive tests and surgical operations.) And so maybe you try to remember that in fact your patient is not necessarily doing this for gain, let alone for pleasure. There may be nothing there that you can find, but that doesn't necessarily make the patient's pain any less real or any less agonizing. It just reflects on the limitations of the medical profession's ability to recognize and diagnose problems, especially problems that don't show up on a blood test or X ray. The patient may well be in very real distress, and his doctor may blame him because the cause of that distress is not detectable with biomedical tests. But it is also true that the doctor may be left worrying, did I miss something?

So if you find the medical student peacefully asleep in a patient bed late one night on the ward, pause to admire her desperation. It wasn't easy to put that IV in her own arm. It wasn't precisely dignified to trade her scrub suit for a hospital johnny that doesn't close in the back and a pair of foam-rubber slippers. She didn't make a sound when they came in to draw blood. Smile down at her gently and ask the nurse to wake her up for her sleeping pill (all the oldest hospital jokes turn out to be simple realism). And, if you are the intern on call, resist the temptation to strike any bargains with the Almighty; you may come down with severe gastroenteritis, but it won't earn you a place in the bed across the hall. You're the doctor.

The Prize in the Cracker Jack Box

"Who is taking care of your baby?"

"Larry. His father."

Over the course of my first summer in the hospital, I perfected a rather pugnacious intonation for that answer, designed to suggest that I would brook no congratulations and no commiseration. I mean, you wouldn't think people would actually imply that you were doing your baby a great disservice by leaving him with his father, would you? And yet some do just that. "Can he take care of such a *little* baby?" they say in hushed tones. Or "That must be really rough for both of them."

I hated it even more when people congratulated me, telling me how lucky I was. There I was, spending altogether too much time in the hospital, missing the baby miserably, missing Larry—not in any mood to be told how fortunate the whole arrangement was. And I always have trouble with people who imply that it's a great stroke of luck that Larry is that mystic entity, that prize in the Cracker Jack box of life, "a good father." I mean, you don't have a baby with someone you think will be a bad father, now do you?

This past summer I spent three months working in the hospital, over a hundred hours a week, every third night on call. My son, Benjamin, was five months old when I started. Larry had the long academic summer

vacation in front of him. It seemed like the right time
for me to get this required three-month stretch out of
the way. I wanted to keep on nursing Benjamin in the
morning and evening on the days I wasn't working
overnight, and I spent the first couple of weeks dash-
ing into hospital bathrooms a couple of times a day to
pull my dress up over my head and express milk,
waiting for my supply to go down to fit the new
schedule.

On the nights I had to stay over in the hospital,
Larry brought the baby to see me at suppertime (I was
supper). When I had a couple of free moments I
would call home and make gooey noises into the phone
for Benjamin and carry on earnest parental conversations with Larry. If an intern or resident whom I
judged less than sympathetic came along while I was
talking, I would switch without warning to highly busi-
nesslike tones: "Okay, thanks for those lab results. I'll
call back later to get the ones that are still pending."

There was an odd sort of parallel between the way
people reacted to me and the way they reacted to
Larry over the summer. Both of us got a lot of com-
ments that sounded like strong (and completely unso-
licited) approval but contained undertones of disap-
proval and even contempt. What I got was "superwoman" nonsense. I was obviously not a candidate for
superwoman; I was a totally frazzled, frequently irritable, chronically sleep-deprived case, depending for my
survival on the support and patience of others—Larry
especially, but also my parents, who got an occasional
hysterical phone call late at night from the hospital.

In any case, many of the compliments I got carried
hostile undertones, implications that I was abandoning
my baby, even that I had selfishly chosen an excitement-
filled summer rather than stay at home: "It must be
nice to be able to throw yourself into medicine now
without worrying about the baby."

What Larry got was gushing praise for being such a perfect new-age father, along with all sorts of unappetizing jargon such as "primary parent" and "role reversal." But frequently there was an undertone there too, and it was, you miserable wimp, how did you ever let yourself get backed into this? What he also received was a constant stream of anxious inquiries: how was he managing, was he able to get through the long days with the baby, could he handle it? Buried in this solicitousness was the constant insulting suggestion that he really didn't know how to take care of a baby.

When Benjamin was born we were both total incompetents when it came to parenthood. You learn fast, of course, and after a couple of months we were quite proficient at all sorts of new skills. It occasionally used to bug me that Larry was always being congratulated for whatever he did with the baby (rock him to sleep, change his diaper), while no one ever congratulated me for any area of competence relative to my new son. There were moments when I really wanted some recognition of how much I had learned— much more, for example, than I ever learned in a comparable period in medical school. During the months right after Benjamin's birth, when I stayed at home, doing my medical courses essentially by correspondence, no one called to ask if I was getting through the long days. There was lots of praise for passing my courses but almost none for caring for the baby. It was a good reminder of how little reinforcement is provided to women who don't work outside the home while their children are small.

The summer went on. Benjamin cut his fourth tooth and was weaned. I became more aggressive about showing pictures of him in the hospital. I tried hard to take care of him when he woke on the nights I was home, and I became very good at snatching one-hour naps in hospital lectures. I worked out rejoinders to remarks about how lucky I was. "Yes," I would say, "and I'm especially lucky to have so much practice getting up at night. The only problem is, the patient spikes a fever, the nurses wake me up, and without a moment's hesitation I diaper the patient." Well, it seemed funny at the time.

By and large, people mean well. One of the lessons of having a baby is that everyone in the world feels free to comment on how you are doing things; strangers come up to you in the street to tell you the baby needs mittens in the wind or the baby is too young to be eating a bagel (Benjamin hates mittens and loves bagels). One of the other lessons of having a baby is that you feel absurdly defensive, anxious to make everyone concede that what you are doing is in fact the one best thing to do ("But the pediatrician specifically recommended that we give him bagels!"). Actually I didn't think this summer that I was doing the one best thing. The arrangement we had was put together out of necessity—the best we could do given a whole variety of constraints.

Now that I have a little time at home I have relearned my baby's daily rhythms and caught up a little on sleep. With a little more distance from the frantic intensity of the summer, I am less irritated by the general need to pass judgment on what I was doing, what Larry was doing. With the attention given nowadays to choices, children and work, men and women (roles and bagels), there is a certain need to make any individual arrangement into a symbol, a case for certain values against others. People feel challenged and defensive about all their most personal familial arrangements and tend to see those of others as either attacking or supporting their own. Many seem to be searching anxiously for both positive and negative models, passing judgment on lives described in newspaper columns and lives lived by colleagues with equal absorption.

When you are privy to the makeshift, catch-as-catch-can quality of your own arrangement, it can be irritating to have people congratulate you on its perfectly-thought-out coordination or else hold you to account for aspects they assume are there by deliberate choice. A little pat on the head is always welcome, of course, especially as you struggle through the difficult times, but you don't actually like to feel that you have been awarded that pat after due consideration by a panel of judges.

Stress and Potato Chips

My journal from last summer, when I worked in the hospital: history sheets meant for patients' records covered instead with disjointed fragments in my most minuscule cramped handwriting. My journal, surrounded by the stern hospital injunctions printed on history sheets: "Enter name and unit number on both sides of every sheet." "Please do not waste space." My journal, written in lectures and conferences, a page of diary hidden beneath a page of conscientious lecture notes—a habit I developed in high school. My journal: endless complaints of fatigue ("worst night in a while, home after no sleep on call and then baby up from 2 to 3 A. M.). Analysis of depression ("The sad truth is, I really want to be doing something I'm good at, and I am just not good at this"). Resolutions ("I have to [1] get more efficient about writing up patients, [2] stop eating potato chips in the middle of the night on call"). Quotes and anecdotes, attempts to record the flavor of the place so I would be able to recall it ("People dying with the TV on, Mr. P. with lung cancer, LA Olympics in the background, swimming races"). And above all, a steady sense of stress, stress so constant and unyielding that I sometimes have trouble recognizing my own familiar voice in my journal.

It will be a long time before my life becomes significantly freer, and even then, it will by no means be without large amounts of strain and complication. Well, I asked for it. I chose this, all of it. I wanted to go to medical school, I wanted to have a baby. I have no real right to complain about the extra sleep-deprivation and emotional weight I lived with over the summer, except perhaps the right to say this: no one can live with that kind of schedule and at the same time do a really good job of being someone's parent. Or a good job of being someone's lover, or someone's spouse, or even someone's close friend. To go through medical training, you have to resign yourself to long periods of time when you will simply do an inadequate job with all the people who mean most to you. And maybe, just maybe, this has something to do with the way many doctors behave when they finish their training, with emotional responses which seem somehow off-key.

Certainly I am not the only medical student who worries about this. At Harvard Medical School graduation ceremonies last June, one of the graduating students made a speech in which he contended that, for him and his classmates, "our careers will not consume our lives." He went on to point out: "The rates of suicide, alcoholism, and drug abuse among physicians— up to eight times higher, maybe more, than among the general population—attest to the toll stress takes on our lives. We want to be more than just good doctors, we want to be good parents and spouses as well."

I look ahead to this life I have chosen with more than a little trepidation. Late at night in the hospital sometimes, we medical students would sit around and half-jokingly analyze all the reasons we were not suited for medicine (I am ideologically opposed to getting up early in the morning, another student says hospitals make his skin crawl, and so on). What we didn't say was that most of us also knew that in some way or other we were people who thrived on stress, performed well under pressure, enjoyed the sense that there would always be more to do than we had time to do, more to learn than we would ever absorb. Certainly I know about myself that I function best when I take on too much, since I have extremely lazy, procrastinating habits. Give me empty time, I waste it. Constant deadlines, extra demands, and I produce. Still, enough is enough.

Over the summer, I found myself envying the people who lived alone. I imagined them returning after a thirty-six-hour stretch in the hospital to quiet, calm apartments, sitting down and staring at the wall for a while, eating or sleeping or going out as they felt inclined. I would come home to Larry and our baby, Benjamin. After long stretches in the hospital I craved domestic pleasures, but they also felt like stresses, further demands on my already strained energy and empathy. I think I felt that if I were going to come home to other people, the least they could do was show sympathy for my weariness, hushed respect for Medicine. Six-month-olds are not strong on hushed respect, of course, and I was left with a kind of ridiculous indignation. As so often in the hospital, I found myself thinking, well, what do they want of me anyway?

Sometimes in my mind, I say to my children, the one who is born and the others I hope to have, "Your mother will be a doctor." And mostly, I feel at least tentatively proud and pleased by that thought. I am still a long way from practicing medicine, but I look through my journal and find the occasional note of jubilation ("Mrs. L. told me she thought I would be a good doctor because I explained her drugs to her so well") and look ahead to a future when the satisfaction, the competence, will come to dominate over the fatigue, the anxiety, the sense of my own ignorance.

As I read through my journal from the summer, I am conscious of an almost desperate clinging to pieces of my own recognizable self, my prejudices about language ("Another lecturer who constantly uses the verb *to share;* gag me with a spoon") and other bits of familiar crankiness. I think about the years ahead, and I suppose that in order to hold onto myself, I will deliberately emphasize my crotchets, the likes and dislikes that were in no way shaped by medical training. I take comfort in that, the idea of a woman in a long white coat, standing, at the end of the next few years, turning up her nose at people who overuse the verb *to share*. Teaching her children to turn up *their* noses ("Your mother is a doctor—and she is also a bit of a pedant"). You get the idea.

I can take comfort in that and, of course, also in smaller things (potato chips in the middle of the night on call, hot-fudge sundaes with Larry and Benjamin off call—so much for good resolutions). And then, as a last resort, I can go to my shelf of totemic books, books that have helped me through all the various pressures and tensions of my life up to this point. And as I try to balance the various things I know I want to do, as I worry about what there will be time for in my life and what will be excluded, I find myself taking comfort from a passage in *Gaudy Night* by Dorothy L. Sayers. Harriet Vane, the heroine, is talking to Miss de Vine, a brilliant scholar:

"But one has to make some sort of choice," said Harriet. "And between one desire and another, how is one to know which things are really of overmastering importance?"

"We can only know that," said Miss de Vine, "when they have overmastered us."

Ignorance

First of all, I want to say that I really do know some things. Really. Or at least some about some things. And I have some useful skills, learned after a good deal of work and a great deal of making a fool of myself—I can start IVs, for example (usually), and handle myself on rounds (often). So I'm not here to confess to absolute blank ignorance.

But as you finish your four years of medical school, it's a little scary to confront the things you don't know. Back in first or second year (depending on how long your naiveté lasted), you could think ahead to the carefully organized, relentlessly studious days when you would finally *put it all together,* learn everything thoroughly and carefully. You could tell yourself that in the clinical years you would finally stop thinking of it all as book learning, and it would begin to make a more immediate kind of sense. Well, yes. And no. People trade little tips back and forth—be sure to do a month of pathology your fourth year; it's a great way to review histology, pathophysiology. . . . Well, maybe it is. But I didn't take it, and neither did many other people.

What I do sometimes (not all the time, really, I promise) is make up little questions that could be directed at me on an oral examination (or in a certain kind of attending rounds). Would you just draw a simple diagram of how the kidney works, and explain what it does? What *is* lymphoma, exactly, and could you outline the various types, symptoms, treatments, prognoses? And so on. How can I not be able to answer questions like that? Oh, I could wing it, use that good old rounds technique, but I couldn't really answer them, not the way you could answer them if you really knew what you were talking about.

In other words, after four years of medical school, I am still waiting to be *found out*. I am still secretly convinced that everyone on my level knows much more than I do—or at least, lots of people on my level. I can't say all of them, because whenever I know someone well, I discover another person afraid of being found out.

You can't know it all. How often we have heard that said to us, but almost always by people who seem to know almost all of it. Still, they were telling the truth; in this business, you can't know it all. And medical students make some of their choices on the basis of how they feel about that; some aim directly for superspecialization, where you can at least know most of what there is to know about your area, and others make their peace with never even approaching knowing it all, and become generalists.

You can't know it all. Like many medical students, I kind of like knowing it all. My response to those nerve-wracking sessions in which I ask myself perfectly reasonable questions I cannot possibly answer thoroughly is to offer myself a different series of questions. I ask myself a list of unfair, picky, highly recherché questions, to which I do happen to know the answers, and I supply the answers in a snidely matter-of-fact tone of voice.

In what disease do you sometimes see purple eyelids?

—Dermatomyositis, of course.

What is the name of the tick that transmits Rocky Mountain spotted fever?

—*Dermacentor variabilis* in this part of the country, *Dermacentor andersoni* farther west.

Now, I have in fact been asked these questions during my medical training, and I remember them as examples of moments when I seemed to shine as someone who might, in fact, know it all, even the little details. Now as it happens, I remember these odd little facts only for odd little reasons; the tick names because I used to be interested in entomology, the purple eyelids because a friend and I once had a running joke about the differential diagnosis of various artifacts—eye shadow, for example. And I should be thankful (and I am thankful) that I wasn't being asked instead for a description of the usual presentation of dermatomyositis, or the typical clinical course of Rocky Mountain spotted fever. By knowing the details, I implied a knowledge of the basics. And that is what roundsmanship is all about—the art of making a good impression on rounds, regardless of what you actually know or don't know.

By the end of their training, medical students know they are pretty safe from those scary basic questions. Your teachers won't ask you how the heart works, they'll ask you some picky question about the latest article in the *New England Journal of Medicine* on cardiac medications. And if you don't know the answer to the question (but you will know it; you learned it last night, because that's what roundsmanship is all about), you'll know how to handle that too, how to offer to go bring in the article in a tone that suggests sincere interest and a profound acquaintanceship with all previous research. That's what roundsmanship is all about.

But just as the further you go along in your training, the safer you are from certain kinds of detection, it is also true that the further you go, the scarier it gets. Not just that it would be even worse to be *found out* as

an intern, but also that you are going to be responsible
for patients, and it is no longer going to be just a
question of trying to do well in school.

But you can't know it all. How do doctors deal with
the certainty of their own ignorance? How do more
senior people, who have spent years caring for patients, acknowledge gaps in their understanding?

When it comes to a collective lack of knowledge,
doctors are understandably more comfortable admitting the gap when only other doctors are present. In
medical school, there was a certain tone in which a
lecturer could say: and we don't know what causes this
and that, we don't know how to treat it, we don't
know what it is. And that tone could often imply, one
of you out there may find it out some day. Sometimes
a lecturer even went so far as to say it: perhaps one of
you will solve this problem.

But talking to patients, doctors are often much stiffer,
much less optimistic, when it comes time to admit we
don't know what causes this. It may even seem as if
the doctor regards this ignorance as a personal lapse,
as if this general lapse has been transformed into the
individual carelessness of a lazy student.

You can't know it all. And even if you knew everything that anyone else knows (which you can't, so stop
worrying about it), you still wouldn't know what you
need to know to help many patients.

I know what I need to do. I need to make my own
ignorance into a constructive force, I need to train
myself to find things out when I don't know them, I
need to train myself out of some of my roundsmanship
habits so I can take advantage of the knowledge of
those who will be supervising me. "Never ask a question on rounds unless you already know the answer," I
was advised early in my clinical training, and you
know what? It's very good advice. If you ask a question on rounds, it usually gets turned back on you, so

asking out of total ignorance makes you look very bad. It is presumably time to unlearn that strategy.

Medical training is not particularly good at helping people to acknowledge their own limitations. Residency, after all, is designed almost without reference to normal human limitations. Medical school does not leave you prepared to deal with patients whom you are powerless to help. Ignorance can seem like the most shameful limitation of all, the one not to be admitted, not to be indulged, above all not to be tolerated. It is the guiltiest of my guilty secrets, and someday I am really going to be *found out*. In order to come to terms with my ignorance, I suppose, I will have to understand that the only one who is going to find me out is the one who already has.

"Who Knows This Patient?"

"Code call, Five South. Code call, Five South." All day the hospital loudspeaker system has been paging one doctor or another, frequently in tones too muffled to be intelligible (was that "Dr. Joe Sung" or "Dr. Johnson"?), relaying messages that suggest small hospital dramas of one kind or another ("Patient Mark Watson, please return immediately to your floor"). All day long people have been listening with a low level of attention, tuned in just enough to catch their own names.

Then "Code call, Five South. Code call, Five South." The operator's voice is the same. No bells ring, no lights flash. But everyone is off and running, pounding down the hall, stethoscopes streaming in the breeze, the resident and the intern running as fast as they can, while you, the medical student, as usual are trailing a tiny bit (just where is Five South anyway, and what would I do if I got there?). A code call means someone has stopped breathing, someone's heart has stopped, someone is dying, come at once.

There's a certain element of competition in the way residents and interns react to a code; you can't "run" the code unless you're one of the early arrivals; if you get there too late, there may well be no role for you. So it's down the stairs two at a time, and you emerge panting on Five South, where you easily locate the room by the crowd of early arrivals massed outside.

The senior medical resident present is running the code, calling out orders. One intern is doing CPR, compressing the patient's chest as he counts, "One-one-thousand, two-one-thousand, three-one-thousand . . ." Another intern is desperately trying to get an IV line started in the patient's arm, while a junior resident is working on putting one into the jugular vein. The patient had only a very small IV in place, and it isn't working well. A respiratory specialist is getting ready to put a breathing tube down the patient's throat. A nurse is taking an electrocardiogram, another is holding an oxygen mask on the patient's face, and others are filling syringes with medicines. Everyone seems purposeful and assured, and although there's a definite air of crisis in the room, there's also a certain calm.

As you stand on the sidelines, you attempt to convey by your demeanor two somewhat conflicting messages: I'm very happy to be of use in any way possible, and please don't give me any responsibility, because I'm terrified. You're a third-year medical student. Most likely, exactly two years ago all these interns were third-year medical students. The residents are another year or two along, but that's all. You aren't watching people who've invested whole careers in learning how to handle this kind of emergency. You're going to be in their shoes in just two years.

When I first started work in the hospital, one of the lectures given to the medical students was about codes. We sat there, remembering all the stories we had been told—"So, they sent this med student to take a patient to X ray, and they got stuck in the elevator and the patient coded right there"—and inventing even worse stories for ourselves. Okay, said the head of our training program, I'm going to teach you how to run a code. Some of us exchanged glances. *Run* a code?

Well, said our teacher, what you do, in order to take control of a code, is stride forcefully into the room, bang on the table, and say fiercely, "Who knows this patient?" Good point—in the chaos of a code it's easy to find yourself caring for a patient without any idea of why that patient is in the hospital in the first place, let alone details like a history of heart attacks or bad lung disease. Anyway, after you've established your authority with that first question, you buttress it by banging on the table again and yelling, "How many amps of bicarb has this patient gotten?" We all laughed—it wasn't serious, we weren't expected to run codes. And then, like many of my fellow students, I carefully wrote down, "Who knows this patient? How many amps of bicarb has this patient gotten?"

There are various terrors tied up with the change from medical student to doctor, but the worst is probably this terror of responsibility. In just a couple of years there will be a life-and-death situation, and you'll be the one making the decisions. And this very dramatic terror serves as a focus for all the vaguer terrors about the other kinds of responsibility in your future, all the small decisions you'll make, all the advice you'll give.

So you stand there, at the code, and imagine yourself as the intern trying to start the IV line. After all, you know how to start an IV. That could easily be you, kneeling at the side of the bed, feverishly swabbing the arm once again with alcohol, searching for a vein. And all you can think is: what if I failed to start it, what if the patient couldn't get the drugs she needed because I never got the IV in?

"Let's give her another amp of bicarb, please," says the senior resident running the code.

Well, by stretching your imagination you can see yourself trying to start the IV, but you certainly can't imagine that you will ever, in a million years, be the one in charge. How can that resident stand there so calmly, even remember to say "please"? How can she be sure she's saying the right things? If it were you, you'd be thumbing desperately through the little spiral-bound outline-of-absolutely-everything you carry in the bulging pocket of your white coat, looking up "code," or "cardiac arrest," or "respiratory failure," or "death."

I remember the first time I saw an intern pull out a similar book and look up what to do. I'd been proceeding miserably along, sure that I was the only one in any way uncertain of my medical knowledge. I watched the intern matter-of-factly look up the instructions for his particular problem, and I felt a tremendous wave of relief—well, if you're allowed to look things up, maybe I might be able to do this too someday. And then I realized that the intern had hurried off to follow the instructions, that he was actually going to *give* the recommended drugs in the dosages he'd just checked, and it suddenly seemed strange and frightening all over again. There's a tremendous gap between looking up what to do so you can say something intelligent when a senior person asks what the right thing to do is, and looking it up so you can then go and do it.

Anyway, the intern has gotten the IV started in the patient's arm. You feel a personal triumph, after identifying yourself so strongly with the attempt. You wait for some congratulations, some recognition, and in fact the senior resident in charge finds a second to say, "Good work." The intern now devotes himself to getting a sample of arterial blood to be analyzed for oxygen content; he's unable to get it from the wrist arteries and has to go for a femoral stick, putting a needle into the major artery in the groin. This is something else you know how to do, and once again you're grateful that you aren't doing it.

*   *   *

The code isn't going well. The patient has been given all the right drugs, the CPR has continued without letup, she finally has a breathing tube in, electric shock to her heart has been tried. She doesn't seem to be responding. You're standing next to the bed of someone you don't know, and she's dying.

The intern gets the arterial blood sample. It looks ominously dark, not the bright red it should be. Finally there's something you can do; the syringe full of blood is put into a cup of ice, and you take it and run down several flights of stairs to the lab, where you puff out that this is a sample from a code. And then you stand there while the technician puts some blood into a machine that will read out the amount of oxygen and carbon dioxide in it. The numbers appear on the meter, and they don't look good. You scribble them down on a piece of paper. The lab will call the patient's floor with the results, of course, but you run back up the stairs and get there before anybody has called.

"Blood gas results," you announce.

"Yes?" The senior resident gives you her full attention. You read the numbers off your slip of paper. The resident reflects for a second, then shakes her head. "They're the same as they were half an hour ago. This woman has essentially been getting no oxygen for half an hour, so in all good conscience I don't think we can continue trying to start her heart up. Her brain will be gone."

There's a pause in the room. Then, slowly, people begin to undo what they've been doing. The electrocardiograph electrodes are removed. The chest compressions stop. All the bustle around the patient's bed quiets down, until just two nurses are left, wiping the patient clean of blood, removing all the various tubes, so that her relatives will see her resting in peace.

"Thank you all," says the senior resident. "Good job."

And as you drift out of the room, you're thinking that you still don't understand how you'll ever make the jump, the assumption of responsibility. After all, it was you who carried those lab values upstairs, you who read aloud the numbers that made the resident decide to stop the code, and that already seems to you a tremendous and terrifying responsibility. And then as you wander down the hall, you catch yourself murmuring under your breath, "Who knows this patient?"

ISSUES

Mr Gibson used to tell him that his motto would
always be "Kill or cure," and to this Mr Coxe once
made answer that he thought it was the best motto a
doctor could have; for if he could not cure the patient,
it was surely best to get him out of his misery quietly,
and at once. Mr Wynne looked up in surprise, and
observed that he should be afraid that such putting
out of misery might be looked upon as homicide by
some people. Mr Gibson said in a dry tone, that for
his part he should not mind the imputation of homicide, but that it would not do to make away with
profitable patients in so speedy a manner; and that he
thought that as long as they were willing and able to
pay two-and-sixpence for the doctor's visit, it was his
duty to keep them alive; of course, when they became
paupers the case was different.

ELIZABETH GASKELL, *Wives and Daughters*

IN THE PREVIOUS SECTION, the general focus of the essays was to convey the sensations as well as the lessons of clinical training. In this next, I want to look at a range of related issues, some of the ethical dilemmas of modern medicine, the problematical areas of the profession. Most are not specific to the training of the medical student, but all are part of this sometimes overwhelming initiation into the hospitals. Some of the essays are very personal, reflecting specific experiences I had—the decision about medication for my own child, the month I spent in an Indian hospital. Others deal with issues that come up in everyone's medical training—seeing a patient labeled DO NOT RESUSCITATE, for example.

Medical education, after all, has to do more than just send you out equipped to deal with a range of diseases. It has to introduce you to some of the touchiest issues around, questions for which there are no answers. And what most of these essays deal with is how it looked, from my perspective as an apprentice.

For some of my clinical training, I have to admit that I wasn't very concerned with ethical niceties. I was trying to keep my own head above water, I was trying to make a good impression, I was trying not to do any damage. But when things relaxed, when I was no longer thinking only in terms of my own survival, then I had to deal with what I had seen and heard, what I was watching and listening to—and doing. Life and death, life-and-death decisions, the decision to limit treatment or to go ahead with a "full-court press," the problem of dealing with deadly infections, or dealing with children in another country who are dying from infections that almost do not exist in my own— all these were also part of my education. And so the essays that follow are in many cases a kind of belated chewing-over of what I experienced.

Many of these experiences are the kind that no doctor ever comes to take for granted. I never met a pediatrician who was at all matter-of-fact about turning off a respirator. Still, as a medical student seeing it all for the very first time, my perspective was probably closer to the perspective of someone outside the profession. And so I hope this section will follow logically from the one before; these are the issues you deal with in the hospital beyond the day-to-day events of sickness and death. These are some of the things you wonder about, when you're finally out of the hospital, trying to think normal, nonmedical thoughts. They aren't all problems of life and death; there is also the question of how, as a doctor, you will get along with your colleagues, the nurses, and a more general question about how power works in the hospital. But all of these issues, how much you think about them and how you think about them, help to shape you as a doctor. They are problems set you by your medical training— not problems set deliberately, and not problems that are susceptible to any simple right answer, but problems all the same. And the answer you provide is the kind of doctor you become.

Power Plays

Oh, someday we too will be attendings, and we will stride through the hospital corridors in the long white coats which are badges of status (even medical students can wear the short white ones) and smile absently at the various peons we pass, the residents and nurses and students and the occasional patient, and we will stride onto the ward and bring order out of chaos, rebuking the house staff (interns and residents) who in ignorance, overeagerness, or sloth (it hardly matters which) have done too little of the right thing or too much of the wrong. We will listen ceremoniously (or is that ceremonially?) to our patients' chests and then reassure them gently that they are in excellent hands—nodding politely to the house staff, but really meaning, of course, ourselves. And we will conduct our formal teaching sessions (attending rounds) and grill the medical students, for their own good, of course, showing them again and again how little they really know, and then when we get tired of the game, we will lecture for a while on our own research interests, and no one will dare fall asleep. (And then we will stride off the ward, making a great show of hurry and importance, and have a nice lunch, and as soon as we are gone, the resident will express himself in scatological terms as regards all emendations made to house-staff management of patients and also as regards attendings who do so much research that they forget what little they ever knew about patient care and, incidentally, say a couple of scathing words to the medical student about a pretty weak showing.) Oh, someday we too will be attendings, and we will have *power*.

Medicine in a large teaching hospital is structured as a rigid hierarchy. The medical student of course is at the bottom; the term "scut-puppy" comes to mind. The hierarchy ascends in order of seniority: the intern, the junior resident, the senior resident, the fellows, the attending. The official expectation is that all doctors will teach medicine to those less experienced than themselves, and that there will also be lessons in the art of being a doctor, in what can be called bedside manner, in all sorts of intangible subjects that can be taught only by example. And one end result is that a lot gets taught and learned about how to handle power.

But wait a minute. Wasn't one group left out of that description of the hospital hierarchy? After all, doctors may flatter themselves that they are the centers of creation (How many Harvard medical students does it take to change a light bulb? One, to stand there and hold it while the world revolves around him), but surely they don't flatter themselves that hospitals exist only for their benefit. Well, no, there are the patients. The patients are outside the hierarchy, but sometimes they can also be found at its most subterranean level, below even the subbasement of the medical students. After all, the lowly medical student often knows more than the patient about the patient's prospects, about possible diagnoses, about tests in the offing, maybe painful or dangerous.

And patient care can be influenced by the issues of power which entangle the various doctors, by the little dramas of territoriality and one-upmanship which sometimes emerge from unfortunate combinations of personalities. Patients can be seen as territory, decisions as power, medical disagreements as personal challenges. An illustrative story, extreme but real:

Mr. Rachmaninoff has been finding himself a little short of breath lately. Of course, he's getting on, and in spite of what he knows about cigarette smoking being bad for your health, he hasn't been able to give up his pack-a-day habit. Otherwise he's in pretty good shape, really, lives alone, does his own shopping, takes the stairs slowly but surely, pays frequent visits to his children and grandchildren. It seems to he a close family; in fact, it's his older daughter who has dragged him to the doctor to have this shortness of breath investigated; Mr. Rachmaninoff has been inclined to write it off as old age. Anyway, as part of the doctor's investigation, a chest X ray is done, and when the chest X ray is read, there is a round lesion in the left upper lobe of the lung. This can mean any number of things, but one of the things it can mean is, of course, lung cancer. And in a gentleman in his late sixties with a heavy smoking history—well, it's worrisome. Mr. Rachmaninoff's doctor decides to admit him to Major University Hospital for fuller investigation of this lesion. For reasons best known to himself, Mr. Rachmaninoff shows up at 10:00 P.M., when the intern on call, who is trying to work up one emergency room admission before she gets hit with the next, is not too happy to see him. As she is rushing down to the emergency room, she runs into the Pulmonary Fellow, who is still in the hospital because it has been an exceptionally busy day, and she remembers that in the note he wrote about Mr. Rachmaninoff, the private physician asked for a pulmonary consultation. So she stops for a minute and tells the Pulmonary Fellow about Mr. Rachmaninoff, and the Fellow, who is young and enthusiastic, says, what the hell, I'll go see the guy now, before I leave. So the intern rushes away, happy, number one, to have fulfilled the request of the pri-

vate physician, and number two, to have gotten someone knowledgeable to see her patient, which will help
her to be on top of the case for the next morning's
rounds.

The Pulmonary Fellow leaves a long note in the
chart. (The intern copies from it extensively for her
own note, which she of course sticks into the chart
before the other note, since hers is the admission note,
and the medical student curses himself for not having
been around when Mr. Rachmaninoff arrived—he was
at the free late-night supper the hospital provides for
people on call, and for the sake of a lousy turkey-loaf
sandwich, he has missed this nice straightforward admission, and the intern will make him do some awful
old emergency room gomer—hospital slang for a very
debilitated, no longer mentally intact patient; stands
for "Get Out of My Emergency Room"—with five
volumes of past medical charts to review and multisystem disease to read up on.) The gist of the Fellow's
note, which learnedly summarizes all the possibilities,
obscure and more obscure, to be considered in the
differential diagnosis of a lesion like Mr. Rachmaninoff's,
is that the Fellow thinks the guy has lung cancer, and
he wants to do a bronchoscopy to prove it—that is,
stick an instrument down the patient's bronchus and
take a biopsy.

The next morning, on work rounds, all hell breaks
loose. The resident is furious at the intern for calling
the consult. Now these Pulmonary guys are gonna
come in and take over *our* patient, and they're gonna
want to make all the decisions. Four or five times he
tells the chastened intern, and her colleague, the other
intern, I don't want you guys calling *any* consults till
you check with me. Got that? *No* consults unless I say
so.

As work rounds are finishing (the resident has just
blown off a little steam by letting the medical student

have it for taking more than ninety seconds to present the patient he worked up, the one with five volumes of old chart and the multisystem disease), the Pulmonary team turns up. With rather elaborately casual intellectual interest, the resident informs them that he is dubious about the value of bronchoscopy in Mr. Rachmanioff's case, and he wants to go with a transtracheal needle biopsy—that is, he wants to stick a needle into the lesion from outside and take a tissue sample that way. The Pulmonary people begin talking about which test is more likely to give definite results with a lesion in this particular location, which test is more dangerous to this patient. There is a rather tense little scene as they and the resident quote journal articles back and forth. Finally the resident, who is not known for his good manners or his subtlety, says, well he's *our* patient and we make the decisions, so tough luck, guys. You don't get to bronchoscope this one.

At attending rounds, the resident tells the story to the attending, casting the Pulmonary Fellows as lawless marauders and the intern as a foolishly ineffectual guard. Now, if the resident is a notoriously bad-tempered would-be cowboy, the attending is deeply concerned with his own diagnostic brilliance, with demonstrating the breadth and depth of his knowledge, with posing questions he can himself answer at length. The attending is roused to furious scorn of the Pulmonary Fellows—why are they so sure this lesion is malignant? (He demands a list of nonmalignant possibilities from the medical student, who has unfortunately fallen asleep, and who wakes up only in time to hear the word "possibilities," spoken with the little interrogative lift which tells him that he has been asked a question. Unfortunately, he guesses the question wrong and begins to list possible types of lung cancer; he is cut off with a few sarcastic words and the attending lists the possibilities he wants himself.) He and the resident are both working themselves up into a fever of hope that they can pull the rug out from under Pulmonary by establishing that Mr. Rachmaninoff in fact has not cancer but tuberculosis (the medical student is told to give him a TB test—a little scut) or some rare fungal infection (the medical student is told to draw blood for a series of antibody tests) or some benign slow-growing kind of tumor (the medical student is told to track down Mr. Rachmaninoff's old chest X rays, which are apparently at a hospital not too far away, so they can be compared with this new one). Mr. Rachmaninoff doesn't know it, of course, but by the time attending rounds are over, he has a large group of doctors cheering for him with a passion no other patient on the floor can even approach. Everyone bustles around, arranging new and different kinds of X rays, hoping to show aspects of the lesion which make malignancy unlikely, drawing blood and ordering more tests, tracking down old chest films and getting radiologists to read them. The Pulmonary people show up in Radiology just as the team is going over these films, and again express a wish to do a bronchoscopy. Absolutely not, says the resident, folding his arms. The intern whispers something apologetic when the resident isn't looking, and the Pulmonary Fellow replies with something short and pointed.

And so it goes on. Unfortunately for the resident and the attending, and even more unfortunately for Mr. Rachmaninoff, none of the benign possibilities pans out. The needle biopsy is attempted without success, and the resident has to allow a bronchoscopy to be done after all—though he makes it clear that he considers it all, including the failure of the needle biopsy, to be the intern's fault for calling in the consult. The bronchoscopy shows that Mr. Rachmaninoff has lung cancer. The attending has changed his tune and begins to insist that he saw it coming all along. He gives a learned little lecture on why lung cancer was always the most likely diagnosis in this patient, and the medical student manages to stay awake and correctly, this time, provide the four possible types of lung cancer when asked.

Mr. Rachmaninoff passes into the hands of the surgeons, who are fighting over whether he is a "surgical candidate"—that is, are his lungs, apart from the cancer, good enough to stand the surgery? And back on the home team, the attending pontificates about how much everyone has learned from this patient, about what good "bread-and-butter medicine" this was, and the resident takes the opportunity to get in a few more digs about people who call in consults and get the patients snatched away from under our noses. And the intern stares straight ahead, and the medical student begins to drift off to sleep. Someday we will be residents. Someday we will be attendings.

Mr. Rachmaninoff, in the end, probably got the same care he would have gotten without the power struggle. Oh, maybe an extra test or two, and certainly a whole lot of extra attention from doctors. He will never know the details of the controversy that raged around his lungs—but of course, from his point of view, he is caught up in a very different and much more serious drama.

Disasters Past

So here we are, a hundred fifty or so medical students in a big lecture hall. The guy who's notorious for doing the *New York Times* crossword puzzle in lecture is doing the *New York Times* crossword puzzle. The guy who's notorious for sleeping with his long legs sprawled onto two seats in the next row is snoring slightly. The five people who are notorious for sitting in the very first row and writing down every single word with their four-color pens are busy clicking from blue to red to green as they try desperately to copy down an extremely complex graph which is flashed on the overhead screen for all of about ten seconds. The rest of us are paying attention, passing notes, drinking sodas, spacing out, looking around the amphitheater to see who is sitting next to whom, paying attention again. And up at the front of the hall is this guy in a long white coat, gesturing with one of those snazzy laser devices that let you point things out with a little red dot. And he's going on about some disease or other, showing slides of graphs and tables and charts and equations. "In a big prospective study . . . various modalities of treatment . . . a control group carefully matched to our patient population for age, sex, race, and ten other relevant variables . . . I think you can see clearly on this graph, though it's a little hard to read from a distance—could we focus, please?"

And then it's as if his tone changes, and suddenly

what he says really comes across: people used to die from this and now they don't have to; this is something we can treat, and treat successfully. And damned if I don't feel a warm, proud glow, second-year student that I am, someone who has never yet touched a real patient. I am a part of that triumphant professional "we," by virtue of my presence in this lecture hall, in this medical school. Somehow, I feel entitled to a tiny bit of the credit for lives saved, pain eased; by starting my medical training, I have joined the long tradition of healing. It's *my* profession too, after all, and I can take personal pride in its accomplishments.

Now, this is all very well, but it's also true that the history of medicine is in part a history of tremendous mistakes, of one-time medical gospels now so thoroughly discredited that it may seem almost unbelievable that anyone ever took them seriously. If we, as beginners, are going to take unto ourselves some of the glory, surely we should also be made aware of the blunders, of the devastating contraventions of what is still the most basic injunction in medicine: "First, do no harm."

Consider, for example, some of the less distinguished moments in the history of obstetrics. There was Dr. Ignaz Semmelweis in the 1850s, trying in vain to convince members of his profession that they could prevent puerperal fever by properly washing their hands after examining diseased cadavers and before examining women who had just delivered babies. He had noticed that the death rates from "childbed fever" were three times as high in the wards where the doctors trained as in those where the midwives worked. And he made the connection: midwives didn't do dissections of cadavers, and so they didn't spread what was called "cadaveric fever." His colleagues didn't take kindly to Dr. Semmelweis's suggestion that they pay attention to their personal hygiene, and it was many years (and many dead women) before his theories were accepted.

Or consider the widespread prescription of thalidomide in the 1950s as a tranquilizer for pregnant women. It isn't pleasant to look back on those doctors, reassuringly prescribing a helpful drug, in all good faith sending women home with the medicine that would deform their children. And then there was DES, a drug originally intended to prevent miscarriage in problem pregnancies, which in some situations was given routinely to all pregnant women, and which has turned out to cause cancer in the offspring of those women. Again doctors threw their professional muscle behind a medicine, and the confidence with which DES was prescribed and overprescribed still disturbingly echoes.

And there it is: if you get to practice medicine with the benign spirits of happy, healthy babies looking over your shoulder, babies who would not have made it without modern medicine, then looking over the other shoulder should be a baby with phocomelia from thalidomide, a twenty-year-old DES daughter with cancer, the ghosts of women who died of physician-transmitted childbed fever. And these images are not stressed in our education. We learn lots of names of doctors who advanced medicine and science, but I find no mention of Dr. Semmelweis in my notes from reproductive medicine. No mention of Dr. Frances Kelsey, the woman in the FDA who virtually single-handedly prevented thalidomide from being marketed in this country—who may have saved some member of my class from being born with the seallike limbs of phocomelia. Somehow, we aren't eager to dwell on these particular heroes of medical science, who tried to save the profession from itself.

As Medicine instructs its neophytes, there seems to be a collective unwillingness to acknowledge fully the disasters of the past, to examine the misuse of that powerful medical authority which can do everything from tell the public what painkiller to buy ("Four out of five doctors surveyed recommend . . .") to cover a sick person with leeches. When I look at my printed lecture notes about thalidomide, I see the heading, "Drugs Taken by Pregnant Women." Am I paranoid to read a subtle message into that phrasing, as opposed to, say, "Dangerous Drugs Sometimes Prescribed for Pregnant Women," or even "Drugs Dangerous to Pregnant Women"? Is there no attempt, perhaps unconscious, to assign the blame away from the medical profession? And then I look a little further on and see a sentence about drugs which are " 'litogens,' drug exposures which have attracted lawsuits in the absence of reasonable scientific data to support cause-effect relationship." And then you sort of have to think back to those doctors who prescribed thalidomide—how did they behave toward patients who asked timidly if it was absolutely safe for the fetus?

I look up DES in my enormous classic medicine text. "It is important to identify the daughters of women who received diethylstilbestrol (DES) during pregnancy. The occurrence of vaginal adenocarcinomas in the offspring of mothers treated with DES during pregnancy demonstrates the problem of detecting carcinogenicity of chemicals."

And somehow all this leaves me wanting more, a fiercer warning, a caution that the medical absolutes we learn and pass on to our patients may turn out to be less than absolute. And that, of course, is the real terror of this refusal to own up to our full professional history. Yes, it is sad and typical that medical school should gloss over reminders of our professional frailty, scare stories which might make us a little humbler and a little more human—qualities not usually high on anyone's personality profile of the typical physician.

But more than that, it's dangerous to refuse to teach the lesson: sometimes the crackpots are right, sometimes the paranoids know what they're talking about. ("The doctor tried to palm off some kind of new medicine on me to help me sleep, but I didn't take it—I knew it was poison for the baby!") Sometimes the awesome weight of medical knowledge is totally off the beam. You have to practice medicine with that in mind, with the knowledge that a hundred years or so along the road, they'll be telling stories about the medical theories of today to get a laugh out of the medical students of 2085—or at least we hope they will. We hope our ways of treating disease will seem merely quaint and improbable to our professional descendants, sitting in lecture, sleeping, doing the *New York Times* crossword puzzle (some things are immortal). We hope that none of our current treatments will turn out to be disastrous horror stories. And then we have to accept the fact that probably some of them will. Who knows what will eventually turn out to be true—pick your own favorite paranoid nightmare. The concerned parent who has read somewhere that vaccinations in childhood may be the cause of immunodeficiency syndromes. The pregnant woman who worries that ultrasound studies during pregnancy result in long-term subtle brain damage and learning disability. Or something so basic, so taken for granted, that no one, not even the pottiest of the crackpots, has gotten around to questioning it. Whatever it is, probably the medical profession is collectively doing something really dumb and really damaging, and doing it with complete goodwill and typical medical self-confidence. And the real question is what their professors will tell those medical students of the future, who, as they sip their futuristic sodas, as they space out and space back in to take a note or two with their ten-color pens (progress is progress), are indeed being initiated into a tradition. And it would be a pity if they were denied knowledge of some of the darker moments in that tradition, denied understanding that the genuine will to heal and help must persist despite fallibility, error, and sometimes disaster.

Nurses

"You want to help sick people?" asks my friend rhetorically. "You want to care for people in pain? Become a nurse." We are both medical students. We are both in the middle of a clinical clerkship on the medical wards of the hospital. What she means is, the nurses spend time with the patients. They get to know them, they meet their families, they tend to their immediate and sometimes desperate needs. They offer comfort, encouragement, explanations. The doctors, with the medical students in tow, show up briefly on morning rounds, returning only if the patient is seriously ill or in need of some procedure or other. When patients leave the hospital, it is the nurses to whom they send thank-you notes, or chocolates, or flowers.

Lewis Thomas, in *The Youngest Science,* writes that he discovered when he was a patient in a big hospital "that the institution is held together, *glued* together, enabled to function as an organism, by the nurses and by nobody else." He also discusses the increasingly adversarial nature of relations between doctors and nurses nowadays.

Why are these relationships so complex? In part, I suppose, because the traditional doctor-nurse relationship was modeled on the traditional male-female relationship; doctors are no longer by definition male, nurses are no longer by definition female, and the relationship between men and women is hardly what it used to be anyway. Nurses, pretty much everyone knows, are overworked and underpaid, and most of all, they aren't accorded a great deal of prestige in the prestige-sensitive medical world. One of the ways that doctors learn to be doctors, it seems, is by learning that they are not nurses and must not stoop to nurses' work.

Evening, and I am sitting at the nurses' station, writing in a patient's chart. I become aware that someone is standing next to me. It is a man I don't know, presumably a patient's relative. "Excuse me, my wife needs a bedpan," he says.

"I'm not a nurse," I respond automatically, pointing out to him a group of nurses.

As he went in search of his wife's nurse, I reflected not for the first time that male medical students (and interns) never get mistaken for nurses, never get asked for bedpans, or dinner trays, or baths. In fact, male nurses sometimes get mistaken for doctors. But a woman in a white coat with a stethoscope around her neck is frequently taken for a nurse.

This can at times be very irritating to those who are insecure about their own status, and as a medical student I was certainly insecure about mine. After all, the medical student's role in the hospital is a little unclear, especially from the patient's point of view. Doctors often introduce medical students as "student doctors," or just as "doctors"—this is contrary to all rules of proper behavior but is done all the time, on the pretext that patients feel more comfortable if they think they are being examined by doctors, no matter how obviously inexperienced. So medical students may feel like frauds.

From their position at the bottom of the pyramid they are keenly aware of their own lack of knowledge, afraid of having their ignorance shown up. So being mistaken for a nurse threatens some pretty shaky egos. The female medical student may even convince herself that by vehemently correcting this mistake, she is striking a blow for women in medicine, and of course in some sense she is: why, when you see a woman in white, do you assume she's a nurse?

Still, nurse or not, why didn't I just get up and get the patient a bedpan if that's what she needed? On the one hand, of course, I was tired—but it wouldn't have taken much time or effort. I suppose it was something that had happened to me during my time in the hospital. At the very beginning of the clerkship, I would have been only too happy to he asked to do something within my capabilities. But now, after a couple of months in the hospital, in some rather mysterious way I had absorbed the various rules and regulations that prescribe what is and is not doctor's work.

I thought back to a story my friend told me early in the rotation. She had helped a patient with his urinal (hospital term for a plastic bottle used by bed-bound male patients) and had been told by two of our (male) fellow students that they would never do such a thing. "I would tell the patient to ring for the nurse."

Other things medical students may consider beneath their dignity: getting a patient a cup of coffee, helping a patient out of his bed and into a chair, cleaning up a mess on the floor. You just tell the patient to ring for the nurse.

There are many tensions built into the relationship between doctors and nurses in the hospital where I was working. The nurses, after all, are there year after year, and the doctors arrive, newly minted each June, and begin telling them what to do. I saw the same page, clipped from a nursing magazine, hanging near nurses' stations all over the hospital. It was a piece that described the two kinds of new doctors nurses have to deal with, the overarrogant and the overtentative.

A medical student who is able to acknowledge the possibility of learning from the nurses' great experience finds them a tremendous resource. The first intravenous line I ever started all alone, I had to start without a doctor standing by. The nurse, who was not allowed to start IVs because of the policy of this particular hospital, but who had started hundreds of them in other jobs, stood across the patient's bed, talking me through it, talking the patient through it.

Nurses are not timid about judging doctors, and one rather sobering experience for a medical student is to get a glimpse of that nursing perspective. Late one night when the intern was busy and I was hanging around the nurses' station, one of the nurses began to point out pictures on a sheet hanging on the wall, meant to identify interns and residents. "Oh yes, we had that one on this floor, he's very arrogant; bad with patients. And that one, she tries to be nice, but she's very intense. Now this one is very good, it was great to have him working here, but that one is a disaster." And so on.

Although experienced nurses know a great deal, and although they are keen judges of budding young doctors and medical students, they are not formally expected to teach us. My first week in the hospital, I asked who was responsible for evaluating my performance. "Oh, everybody," I was told. "Everybody? You mean, interns, residents, and nurses?" The reply was, "Well, not nurses, of course." Of course.

It's sad that the hospital system divides its workers so rigidly that large reservoirs of knowledge and understanding are lost. It wouldn't do a medical student any harm to see the hospital from the point of view of a nurse (or from that of a patient, for that matter, as Lewis Thomas did). But nurses do not

teach in medical school. Instead we are taught by
doctors, the people we will eventually become, and
we absorb their perspective as we struggle toward
their title.

Baby Poop

There are a million stories in the naked city, and some of them are about baby poop. I'm sorry, I try to keep these hospital anecdotes I tell relatively uncrude, but hospitals are hospitals, and sometimes things do get a little bit graphic. But bear with me, because this particular story is fraught with meaning.

Well, there we were on the neurology consult team, a senior attending neurologist, a resident in the neurology program, a resident in the general pediatrics program who was doing a month of neurology, and two medical students, one of them me. And we got called down to the newborn nursery to do a neurological exam on a baby. And we strode in, a phalanx, our reflex hammers peeking from our pockets. We wrapped ourselves in clean hospital gowns and regrouped around the bassinet holding the baby in question, ready to bring all our different levels of expertise to bear on the problem.

I looked down at the baby. My years as a mother have trained me in certain rapid diagnostic methods. I sniffed the air over the bassinet. "This baby is poopy," I announced to the assembled doctors. "He needs to be changed."

No one acknowledged my statement, and I realized that in allowing my private life to contribute to my hospital work, I had used the wrong vocabulary. I tried again. "This baby has apparently had a bowel movement," I said. "Let me just put a clean diaper on him."

This time I got a response. No, no, said all the doctors. They shook their heads, they motioned to me not to bother. Don't change him. We'll just do our exam, and then the nurses will take care of it.

Well, after all, I was only a lowly medical student. So I nodded, and we turned our attention to the neurological examination. We shined lights in the baby's eyes, we tapped for reflexes. We picked him up and held him in the air to assess his muscle tone. We discussed what we thought we saw. We repeated any doubtful tests. In all, we stood around that bassinet for a good forty minutes.

Now, at the risk of making this story even cruder, I have to point out that the atmosphere around that bassinet was really not very pleasant. I mean, you didn't have to be an expert parental type to detect the contents of that diaper. What I mean is, that baby smelled. I mean stank. I mean, even in the hospital, I have been in pleasanter places for forty minutes. But none of us admitted in any way that there was anything to smell except the standard aroma of disinfectant. We stood tall. We were doctors. We did not hold our noses. And finally we finished our exam and marched out; as we left the room, a nurse came hurrying over to the bassinet, carrying a paper diaper.

I have to admit, this is one of my very favorite doctor stories. I have told it several times, and it has elicited a couple of responses I hadn't counted on. So first of all, I want to tell you my interpretation of the story, the interpretation I was forming as I stood by that bassinet. And then, I want to turn the story inside out a couple of times, to suggest other meanings.

I stood by that bassinet, thinking, I cannot believe this. I wasn't so much concerned for the baby—as far as I can tell, small babies are not nearly as eager to have their diapers changed as their parents are to do the changing. But I couldn't believe this group of doctors was choosing to spend forty minutes in this poopy ambience, when thirty seconds of work with a paper diaper would have taken care of the problem.

It occurred to me that perhaps the doctors were squeamish about seeing a diaper changed. I didn't know for sure that any of them had children of their own, and I have encountered people before who imagine that the changing of a diaper is a lengthy and profoundly disgusting process. But still, I reminded myself, these men were *doctors*. They had dissected cadavers, put in their time in the operating room, coped with all the sounds and sights and smells of the hospital. They ought to be able to take it, I thought; they won't faint at the sight of baby poop.

Well, that wasn't really what it was about, I knew. What it was about was dignity. *Doctors don't change diapers*. That's all there was to it; I had offered to do a job that would have compromised my professional status, and by extension theirs, since I was on the same career path as they. I don't mean to suggest they had actually thought it through; I think it was the instinct of professional self-defense that prompted their response. Probably at home they would have changed a baby's diaper—maybe one or two of them had children at home and changed diapers all the time, I didn't know. I'm not sure it would have made any difference; the business executive who at home is fully capable of answering the phone will sometimes let it ring forever in the office if the secretary isn't there. Part of prestige is the jobs you do; the other part is the jobs you don't do. And the strong smell of baby poop is better than a whiff of cleaner air from lower down the totem pole.

So that was the conclusion I reached as we stood in

the newborn nursery. That to me was the point of the
story: in my naivete as a medical student, allowing my
parental responses to take over, I had made a suggestion which was incompatible with doctorly dignity. I
thought it was funny because it was so indicative of the
flip side of dignity, the pompous determination to
preserve prestige at any cost, even if the prestige you
preserve only makes your life unpleasant. I would
have told the story with a punch line something like
this: doctors—they'll save the baby's life, but they
won't change the baby's diaper.

So I told the story, and a gentleman who is a professor of philosophy promptly informed me that if this
had happened in his department, he and his colleagues
would have prevented me from changing the baby too.
I will leave aside the question of how it could have
happened in his department; I have never studied
philosophy and so have no idea what goes on behind
those doors. Anyway, he told me, if there had been a
baby who needed changing, and if I, the only woman
in the room, had offered to do it, they would never
have let me. Even if all the male philosophers had
been unwilling or unable to diaper that baby, they
would not have permitted me to do the dirty work. It
would have looked too much like making the woman
do the woman's work, he explained to me. It was too
sensitive an issue; people were too self-conscious about
it. My immediate response to this was that doctors
were certainly *not* too self-conscious about it—I had
no fear that they had stopped me for such politically
advanced reasons. I suppose you could argue in fact
that just the opposite was going on; as a doctor-to-be,
I was "elevated" to the status of an honorary male. Or
at least, I had joined the traditionally male profession,
and they were not about to let me demean it with

women's work; the diaper was changed by a nurse, a woman doing a woman's job.

Again, I don't mean that any of those doctors actually thought this through. I just mean that the political dynamic that was operating around that bassinet was in fact the traditional dynamic of sexual differentiation.

But when I thought further about this philosopher's comment (still resisting the temptation to imagine what the poopy baby might have been doing in the philosophy colloquium in the first place), it occurred to me that in fact my willingness to change the baby's diaper had something to do with my own attitudes toward the sexual politics of medicine. A year earlier, I'm not sure I would have offered. When I first started out in the hospital, I wouldn't have offered, simply because I never offered to do anything unless I was sure it was my place. If none of the doctors had mentioned it, I wouldn't have either; I would have been worried that perhaps my diaper-changing technique was not smooth enough to show off in front of an attending. And then, after I got over those first-time jitters, I went through a period in which I was very sensitive about sexism. I worried that if I did anything that marked me too distinctly as female, I would be respected less. I resented being mistaken for a nurse. I didn't talk much about my own child. When I wanted to leave the hospital a little bit early to meet his day-care teacher, I said I wanted to go over to the medical school library to look up some articles. When some doctor complimented me on my knowledge of the pediatric dosage schedule of a particular antibiotic, I didn't say, my kid takes that when he gets an ear infection.

But I got over most of this nonsense. By the time I met the baby in my story, I think I had honestly come to believe that both my experiences as a woman and my special skills as a parent add something to my abilities as a doctor. Being able to diaper a baby (and being willing to diaper a baby) is a skill, and a skill it is better to have than not to have. I offered to diaper that baby because I wasn't worried that 1 was being pressured into doing it because I was a woman; I offered to do it because I knew I could do it and I wanted the baby to be wearing a clean diaper. And if anyone had made any cracks about female doctors, I would have despised him, and not myself. It's not a very high peak to have scaled, but I'm glad to have attained that vantage point.

Well, so much for my various kinds of arrogance: the medical student who sees through the doctors, the woman who sees through the men, the sensitive human being who sees through everyone. I told this story one more time, to someone who is not a doctor and not a professor of philosophy. She heard me through to the end, smiled but didn't laugh, and then asked, in a worried tone of voice, "Was the baby okay?"

"What do you mean?" I asked, thinking that sitting around in a poopy diaper for a while never really hurt anyone.

"You were called to do a neurological exam on a newborn baby, you said. Was the baby okay?"

What can I say? Isn't that obviously the right question to ask? Isn't that the detail I completely omitted from my story? Did it in fact occur to me as relevant, when I was doing my cute imitation of the doctors standing around the bassinet, inhaling baby poop? In fact, this particular baby was fine, or at least we couldn't find anything wrong with him, though we spent forty minutes trying. I can't remember what had originally made them suspicious that he was not neurologically intact, but whatever it was, he seemed to have gotten over it. But the fact is, I would probably still have thought I had a good story if the baby hadn't been okay. Someone else had to hear the story to point out to me that actually I and all the other doctors were peripheral characters. And when I was congratulating myself on my ability to escape the doctor's perspective, just because I offered to change the diaper, I was in fact as caught up in my own performance as any of those doctors.

One in Ten Thousand

"Actually, you Yanks aren't using this drug at all anymore," the British doctor said, as he wrote out my prescription. "You've been scared off by the side effects." He chuckled as he passed the slip of paper across to me, and I smiled back, a little bit weakly.

I had just spent a month in London, working as a visiting medical student at the Hospital for Tropical Diseases. I had brought my little family along and we had sublet a place near Kensington Gardens. Larry had been doing the London museums with the systematic enthusiasm of an academic, and our son, Benjamin, eighteen months old, had fed the ducks in Hyde Park every day, rain or shine (mostly rain). We had planned to do some traveling after the month was over, and had been influenced by the people I saw every day at the hospital, returning from one exotic country after another. There were cheap flights out of London to every city in Asia. We would fly to Bangkok, we decided, and spend three weeks in Thailand and Burma.

So I went to one of the pleasant doctors with whom I had been working; I had seen them advise many people who were about to set off into the unknown. We all got our various shots. (I was okay. The baby was fine. Larry is a chicken.) And then I asked about malaria prophylaxis and was given the same advice I had heard plenty of British travelers get: take chloroquine and Fansidar. And then he wrote out the Fansidar prescription for me after we had worked out the baby's dose, and while he was writing it he made the comment about the side effects.

A little later on, I brought it up again, speaking in a casual medical-student-requests-information-for-intellectual-satisfaction voice. Oh, said the doctor, equally casually, you know, Fansidar has been linked to Stevens-Johnson syndrome—I believe there have even been a couple of deaths, so your Center for Disease Control is recommending against it. That's all. But it's the best drug we have, I prescribe it all the time. I've taken it myself.

What does the medical student do now? Admit that she doesn't actually remember what Stevens-Johnson syndrome is? Well, no; I had some misguided idea that every time I confessed some new point of ignorance, they were all shaking their heads at the barbarous ignorance of the whole American medical profession. I kept quiet and went to the library and looked it up. Very reassuring; severe erythema multiforme with involvement of the mucous membranes, sometimes of the respiratory system . . .

The next day at the hospital, I asked, again just-as-a-matter-of-academic-curiosity, how frequently Fansidar caused this response. No one was sure, and no one was terribly interested. I got another little speech about the tendency of America to go overboard, panic, throw out a valuable drug because of some rare side effects. I had heard this before; it went with the jokes about CAT scans which would be made whenever a patient came into the hospital with a straightforward diagnosis. "I suppose you'd get a CAT scan back in Boston, wouldn't you?" one of the doctors would say to me, as we considered the case of a man with a positive skin test for tuberculosis, a chest X ray showing apical consolidations, and a history of night sweats, fevers, and hematemesis—all the textbook signs of TB.

Anyway, it occurred to me as I wandered around the hospital, feeling the spleens of patients with various types of malaria, that in all the times I had seen Fansidar prescribed to travelers setting off for Asia or Africa, I had never heard any doctor talk about fatal side effects. I had been handed this extra information because I was a medical student, and I had been handed it in the spirit of an-interesting-fact-you-might-like-to-know. Many of the doctors at that hospital prescribed Fansidar as the best possible drug for people traveling to certain countries, and saw no reason to dwell on rare and unpreventable reactions, any more than an American doctor in the emergency room feels the need to go into detail about irreversible aplastic anemia before starting a child on chloramphenicol for a suspected bacterial meningitis. Furthermore, it would never have occurred to any of the doctors at the Hospital for Tropical Diseases to suggest that we rethink our trip, change our destination. Their lives revolved around trips to the tropics; most of their families had been on and off malaria prophylactics for years. Of course you go to the tropics, and of course you take the best drug possible.

But because I was a medical student, they had gone out of their way to make my life complicated, I thought resentfully (ignoring the fact that if I had been a better-informed medical student, I would have known the risks of Fansidar for myself). And here I was with a full-fledged moral dilemma: was I going to give my child a medicine with a potentially fatal side effect? Me, I would take it without hesitation; we all have our areas of bravery and our areas of fear, and while I do not dive into swimming pools, and dislike automobiles, I do not mind small planes and dubious airlines,

and I don't worry about rare drug side effects. And
Larry is a chicken about shots but was perfectly willing
to take Fansidar. But did we have any right to give it
to our baby just so we could satisfy our longing to see
the pagodas of Southeast Asia and investigate Thai
food in its native form? More seriously, we weren't
scared for ourselves, but we were terrified for Benjamin. But how big was the danger? What about all
those tourists and students of Buddhism and church
group volunteers and engineering company employees
with families, all those people whom I saw take their
Fansidar prescriptions and walk happily away to get
them filled? This is so unfair, I kept thinking, none of
them have to deal with this decision. Why me?

And the answer of course was that it was completely
fair. I was on my way to being a doctor; this decision I
was being asked to make for my own child was a
decision I would in the future make for other people's
children, and without prolonged agony, either. I had
to evaluate the unavoidable risk involved in a thera-
peutically valid medication, and then balance that
against all the reasons to incur or avoid the risk. In a
way, it was just another one in the unending series of
parental decisions: shall we take our baby to London
for a month (a relative calls up to warn of airline
crashes and IRA bombs)? how about to Thailand and
Burma? shall we let our baby ride for five minutes in a
taxi without a car seat? shall we let our baby kiss that
dog? But it was also a decision with obvious and
specific parallels for my future in medicine: shall I give
this drug? As a medical student finishing my third
year, I had never actually had that responsibility all to
myself before. I had been allowed to suggest drugs, to
offer my opinion, but someone senior had always had
to okay it—and a good thing, too. But there I was in
London with the full authority to decide whether or

not to give my son Fansidar. The decision was too
much for me; I panicked.

After calm and cool reflection, in my case marked
by eating my nails and also a large quantity of tandoori
chicken, I decided to call the Center for Disease Control in Atlanta. A pleasant doctor spoke with me at
length—again, because I was a medical student, he
assumed I would be interested in all the ramifications
of the Fansidar controversy. They had twenty-three
cases of serious reactions documented, with seven
deaths, giving a fatality rate less than or equal to one
out of every ten thousand people who took the drug—
the exact statistic varied according to what method
was used to estimate the total number of people taking
Fansidar. No, this doctor finally said to me, he would
advise against our taking it, against giving it to the
baby. Better to go and risk getting malaria, which is a
treatable disease.

But even in a baby? I asked, remembering what I
heard a doctor say at the Hospital for Tropical Diseases: I've seen cerebral malaria in an infant present
as grand mal seizures, followed by death.

Well, said the doctor in Atlanta, to tell the truth, I
think you're being very irresponsible to take your baby
into a malarial zone. It's your decision, of course, but
if I were you I would just stay home.

Well, there it was. Useless to protest that I had seen
all sorts of people with all sorts of children sent off
into the tropics without being told they were crimi-
nally irresponsible. I was a medical student, I was
expected to know the risks and weigh the risks with
something beyond parental responsibility. Useless to
argue that there were all kinds of risks my child
didn't take—we have no car, for example, while
other children are daily exposed to the dangers of
the highway.

I was caught between my future as a doctor and my past. I was afraid to make a decision because I had never made such a decision. But I was being asked to make it only because I would in fact soon be a doctor, responsible for making many such decisions. But I wasn't a doctor yet, and I was too ignorant and terrified to jump the gun. I didn't want to go forward. I couldn't go backward. So I went round and round.

Well, we went to Thailand and Burma. I want to work with tropical diseases someday—that's how I got to London in the first place. I can't adjust to considering large pieces of the world off limits, and I guess I also accept that my occupation may put certain risks on my family, as it would if I were a diplomat or a police officer. Which is a self-serving way of saying that I wasn't willing to rule out exotic travel as unsafe; I don't drink, I don't ski, I don't drive, but I do travel. And I do rationalize.

We went to Thailand and Burma, and we took the Fansidar. It might have made sense for Larry and me to hold off and run the risk of malaria, but if we were going to give the pills to our baby, we were going to take them too. And of course we were all fine. And since then I've read more about the drug, and frankly, I might decide differently if I had to do it again. And so what? Well, we were lucky, and everything worked out well, and we didn't get hijacked and we didn't get diarrhea, and we didn't get erythema multiforme. But the decision, with its acceptance of risks, was real for all that. And it's just as real that I'll have to make many such decisions in the coming years. I don't exactly know if there's any way to learn to make decisions like these, or to prepare yourself for the time when the luck goes against you. I do know that I will never order a drug with potentially serious side effects, however necessary the drug, without thinking, even for a split second, about the days when I looked down at my own child and thought about Fansidar.

India

The people look different. The examining room is crowded with children and their parents, gathered hopefully around the doctor's desk, jockeying for position. Everyone seems to believe, if the doctor gets close to *my* child everything will be okay. Several Indian medical students are also present, leaning forward to hear their professor's explanations as they watch one particular child walk across the far end of the room. I stand on my toes, straining to see over the intervening heads so I, too, can watch this patient walk. I can see her face, intent, bright dark eyes, lips pinched in concentration. She's about ten years old. I can see her sleek black head, the two long black braids pinned up in circles over her ears in the style we used to call doughnuts. All she's wearing is a long loose shirt, so her legs can be seen, as with great difficulty she wobbles across the floor. At the professor's direction, she sits down on the floor and then tries to get up again; she needs to use her arms to push her body up.

I'm confused. This patient looks like a child with absolutely classic muscular dystrophy, but muscular dystrophy is a genetic disease carried on the X chromosome, like hemophilia. It therefore almost never occurs in girls. Can this be one of those one-in-a-trillion cases? Or is it a more unusual form of muscle disease, one that isn't sex-linked in inheritance?

Finally the child succeeds in getting up on her feet,

and her parents come forward to help her dress. They pull her over near to where I'm standing, and as they're helping with the clothing, the long shirt slides up over the child's hips. No, this isn't one of those one-in-a-trillion cases. I've been watching a ten-year-old boy with muscular dystrophy; he comes from a Sikh family, and Sikh males don't cut their hair. Adults wear turbans, but young boys often have their hair braided and pinned up in those two knots.

Recently I spent some time in India, working in the pediatric department of an important New Delhi hospital. I wanted to learn about medicine outside the United States, to work in a pediatric clinic in the Third World, and I suppose I also wanted to test my own medical education, to find out whether my newly acquired skills are in fact transferable to any place where there are human beings, with human bodies, subject to their range of ills and evils.

But it wasn't just a question of my medical knowledge. In India, I found that my cultural limitations often prevented me from thinking clearly about patients. Everyone looked different, and I was unable to pick up any clues from their appearance, their manner of speech, their clothing. This is a family of Afghan refugees. This family is from the south of India. This child is from a very poor family. This child has a Nepalese name. All the clues I use at home to help me evaluate patients, clues ranging from what neighborhood they live in to what ethnic origin their names suggest, were hidden from me in India.

The people don't just look different on the outside, of course. It might be more accurate to say *the population is different*. The gene pool, for example: there are some genetic diseases that are much more common here than there, cystic fibrosis, say, which you have to keep in mind when evaluating patients in Boston, but which would be a show-offy and highly unlikely

diagnosis-out-of-a-book for a medical student to suggest in New Delhi (I know—in my innocence I suggested it).

And all of this, in the end, really reflects human
diversity, though admittedly it's reflected in the strange
warped mirror of the medical profession; it's hard to
exult in the variety of human genetic defects, or even
in the variety of human culture, when you're looking
at it as a tool for examining a sick child. Still, I can
accept the various implications of a world full of different people, different populations.

The diseases are different. The patient is a seven-
year-old boy whose father says that over the past week
and a half he has become more tired, less active, and
lately he doesn't seem to understand everything going
on around him. Courteously, the senior doctor turns
to me, asks what my assessment is. He asks this in a
tone that suggests that the diagnosis is obvious, and as
a guest I'm invited to pronounce it. The diagnosis,
whatever it is, is certainly not obvious to me. I can
think of a couple of infections that might look like
this, but no single answer. The senior doctor sees my
difficulty and offers a maxim, one that I've heard
many times back in Boston. Gently, slightly reprov-
ingly, he tells me, "Common things occur commonly.
There are many possibilities, of course, but I think it is
safe to say that this is almost certainly tuberculous
meningitis."

Tuberculous meningitis? Common things occur commonly? Somewhere in my brain (and somewhere in
my lecture notes) "the complications of tuberculosis"
are filed away, and yes, I suppose it can affect the
central nervous system, just as I can vaguely remember that it can affect the stomach and the skeletal
system. . . . To tell the truth, I've never even seen a
case of straightforward tuberculosis of the lungs in a

small child, let alone what I would have thought of as a rare complication.

And hell, it's worse than that. I've done a fair amount of pediatrics back in Boston, but there are an awful lot of things I've never seen. When I was invited in New Delhi to give an opinion on a child's rash, I came up with quite a creative list of tropical diseases, because guess what? I had never seen a child with measles before. In the United States, children are vaccinated against measles, mumps, and rubella at the age of one year. There are occasional outbreaks of measles among college students, but the disease is now very rare in small children. ("Love this Harvard medical student. Can't recognize tuberculous meningitis. Can't recognize measles or mumps. What the hell do they teach them over there in pediatrics?")

And this, of course, is one of the main medical student reasons for going to study abroad, the chance to see diseases you wouldn't see at home. The pathology, we call it, as in "I got to see some amazing pathology while I was in India." It's embarrassing to find yourself suddenly ignorant, but it's interesting to learn all about a new range of diagnoses, symptoms, treatments, all things you might have learned from a textbook and then immediately forgotten as totally outside your own experience.

The difficult thing is that these differences don't in any way, however tortured, reflect the glory of human variation. They reflect instead the sad partitioning of the species, because they're almost all preventable diseases, and their prevalence is a product of poverty, of lack of vaccinations, of malnutrition and poor sanitation. And therefore, though it's all very educational for the medical student (and I'm by now more or less used to parasitizing my education off of human suffering), this isn't a difference to be accepted without outrage.

The expectations are different. The child is a seven-month-old girl with diarrhea. She has been losing weight for a couple of weeks, she won't eat or drink, she just lies there in her grandmother's arms. The grandmother explains: one of her other grandchildren has just died from very severe diarrhea, and this little girl's older brother died last year, not of diarrhea but of a chest infection. . . . I look at the grandmother's face, at the faces of the baby's mother and father, who are standing on either side of the chair where the grandmother is sitting with the baby. All these people believe in the possibility of death, the chance that the child will not live to grow up. They've all seen many children die. These parents lost a boy last year, and they know that they may lose their daughter.

The four have traveled for almost sixteen hours to come to this hospital, because after the son died last year, they no longer have faith in the village doctor. They're hopeful, they offer their sick baby to this famous hospital. They're prepared to stay in Delhi while she's hospitalized, the mother will sleep in the child's crib with her, the father and grandmother may well sleep on the hospital grounds. They've brought food, cooking pots, warm shawls because it's January and it gets cold at night. They're tough, and they're hopeful, but they believe in the possibility of death.

Back home, in Boston, I've heard bewildered, grieving parents say, essentially, "Who would have believed that in the 1980s a child could just die like that?" Even parents with terminally ill children, children who spend months or years getting sicker and sicker, sometimes have great difficulty accepting that all the art and machinery of modern medicine are completely helpless. They expect every child to live to grow up.

In India, it isn't that parents are necessarily resigned, and certainly not that they love their children less. They may not want to accept the dangers, but poor people, people living in poor villages or in urban slums, know the possibility is there. If anything, they may be even more terrified than American parents, just because perhaps they're picturing the death of some other loved child, imagining this living child going the way of that dead one.

I don't know. This is a gap I can't cross. I can laugh at my own inability to interpret the signals of a different culture, and I can read and ask questions and slowly begin to learn a little about the people I'm trying to help care for. I can blush at my ignorance of diseases uncommon in my home territory, study up in textbooks, and deplore inequalities that allow preventable diseases to ravage some unfortunate populations while others are protected. But I can't draw my lesson from this grandmother, these parents, this sick little girl. I can't imagine their awareness, their accommodations of what they know. I can't understand how they live with it. I can't accept their acceptance. My medical training has taken place in a world where all children are supposed to grow up, and the exceptions to this rule are rare horrible diseases, disastrous accidents. That is the attitude, the expectation I demand from patients. I'm left most disturbed not by the fact of children dying, not by the different diseases from which they die, or the differences in the medical care they receive, but by the way their parents look at me, at my profession. Perhaps it is only in this that I allow myself to take it all personally.

When Doctors and Patients Speak Different Languages

The attending is interrogating the patient's parents, snapping out questions in rapid Hindi. Well, not the attending, the *consultant;* the nomenclature in Indian hospitals follows the British system, and what we in the United States call an attending, they call a consultant. Anyway, the consultant has assumed a rather aggressive manner toward these two parents; he asks the same question over and over until he is satisfied with their answers. The patient, a one-year-old boy who is about the size of a healthy six-month-old, is sound asleep in his mother's arms, well wrapped in a shawl as it is chilly by local standards (about seventy degrees outside right now and everyone's wearing at least one heavy sweater).

We crowd around the desk and lean forward to listen to the interrogation, twelve Indian medical students and I. They, of course, can understand what is being said; I am left listening to the tones of voice, catching the not infrequent cognates, and waiting for translation. Actually, though, the mother's voice has now sunk so low that her replies are not audible from across the desk.

The consultant is finally satisfied. He looks away from the couple with the child and announces in English to the group of medical students: "You see, finally we have the true story. They stopped breast-feeding the child at the age of six months, and imme-

diately they started feeding him with this expensive
canned formula. But when you ask in detail, how
many spoonfuls of formula, it turns out they don't
have enough money, so they have been diluting it."
He pauses. "They keep repeating the name of the
formula because they are so proud that it is an expensive brand, whereas in fact they are starving their child
to death. And they have already lost one child, in this
same exact way."

Throughout this speech, the two parents look from
the consultant to the medical students, back and forth,
searching for some clue to what is being said, to how
their son is being assessed. But the consultant's tone is
calm, the medical students are scribbling in their note-
books, and the parents are left to wait, hoping for a
translation.

In the great globe-hopping tradition of the fourth-
year medical student, I was working in the clinic of a
major teaching hospital. All instruction of medical
students and house staff, all lectures and seminars,
and most conversations between doctors took place in
English. Medical students scribbled their notes in English and presented their cases in English—and very
formal English, too, beginning each statement with
"sir" or "ma'am," according to the sex of the consultant ("Sir, this is a one-year-old boy who presents with
a complaint of small size and failure to grow"). Hospital records were also kept in English. But communica-
tions between doctors and patients took place in Hindi,
because, except in very unusual cases, the patients
spoke little or no English.

For the first few days, I found it very strange to
have doctors calmly making, in front of patients, such
statements as, "They are starving their child to death."
Because it was a teaching hospital, the consultant often had a point to make about history-taking, might
want to indicate a dubious fact or two. Or the consul-

tant might be assessing the socioeconomic status of the patients: "These are very poor, uneducated people, who have not followed the instructions we gave them last time."

As I say, I found this very strange, this matter-of-fact way of discussing a patient in that patient's presence, perhaps assigning blame to parents, perhaps doubting the accuracy or honesty of a history, perhaps even speculating as to prognosis—all in the patient's hearing, but in a language the patient did not speak. It seemed to reinforce the rigidity of the class divisions in the hospital, members of the middle class (English-speaking) caring for members of the lower class (non-English-speaking). It seemed callous and a tiny bit surreal, like an actor stopping mid-scene for an aside to the audience that all the other actors are apparently unable to hear.

In fact, it was really none of those things. The ability to speak English is indeed a tool for professional advancement, and it is absolutely required of medical students. It was neither callous nor surreal, it was simply a convention of medical education. And the interesting thing was that after a few days in this environment, it had come to seem quite familiar to me. I had adjusted myself to the rather dramatic change from Hindi to English and had come to see it as a parallel to the change doctors make back home, the change from speaking to a patient in normal people-talk, to discussing that patient in medical jargon.

Would a doctor in the United States say in front of parents, "They are starving their child to death"? Well, I hope not. Might a doctor (or a medical student, presenting at the bedside) say, "This seems to be a case of nonorganic failure to thrive secondary to inadequate caloric intake with possible psychosocial roots"? Well, maybe. Or something like that. And heaven knows it's possible to speculate about diagnosis and

even prognosis so that the patient has no real understanding of what is being discussed. In fact, I realized I
had seen that same uncertain, lost look on the faces of
patients at home in Boston, the look that was really an
appeal for a translation. And then that same shifting
of gears as the doctors turned back to the patient to
explain, "What we've just been saying is . . ."

Over the past couple of years, I have grown very
accustomed to this kind of switching back and forth; I
think medical students often err, at the beginning of
their clinical training, in one direction or the other. It
is the stuff of which medical student jokes are made,
on the simplest levels; the medical student who ner-
vously asks a patient, "Have you had any diplopia?"
or who says cheerfully to an attending, "Review of
systems is positive for getting sick to his stomach."
And so, as you progress through the clinical training,
it gradually becomes second nature to use the right
words, expressions, patterns of speech with attendings
and other physicians, and then recover normal human
speech to use with patients, or else create a new and
slightly artificial jargon for patients. And this division
becomes a vital element in your emerging professionalism; you can communicate with doctors as a doctor,
and then switch over and speak to a patient in a
language that is no longer necessarily your native
tongue.

We are on rounds in New Delhi, pausing at the
bedside of a child in a coma from tuberculous meningitis. For weeks he has been rceiving antituberculous
drugs; the neurosurgeons have already put in a shunt.
Gently, in Hindi, the consultant questions the child's
father, who has been sleeping in the hospital, washing
and caring for his son. The mother and the four other
children are in a distant home village; the doctors have
already tried hard to convince this man that when he
returns home, he must take his whole family to be

tested for TB. He agrees, but right now he can see no farther than his silent, motionless son. The consultant is asking whether the father has seen any changes in the child over the past couple of days, any responsiveness to speech or light, any movements. (Nursing care is limited, so the father is the only one to ask for this information.) No, the father is saying, no change, no response to anything, no movement.

The consultant turns to the group of house staff and medical students. "We are getting close to the cutoff point, I think," he says. "We will have to make the decision very soon to stop giving any more drug therapy unless we see some changes, and I very much doubt that we will."

The father listens intently to the doctor's words, trying perhaps to draw some hope from the tone of voice, trying perhaps to guess what decisions are being discussed. I can't help wondering: if he knew what was being said, would he lie to us, tell us his son was improving? would he try to buy a few more weeks of drug therapy, hope no one would check his claims? I don't know, of course, what he would do. And he doesn't know, of course, what we are talking about. He doesn't speak our language.

AIDS

The patient has AIDS. Therefore, in obedience to the signs posted on this door, we are putting on gloves and masks. Finally we troop into his room and stand around his bed, our faces obscured by surgical masks, our hands encased in plastic skins. The resident looks down at the sick man in the bed, and suddenly sounds a little abashed. "Um, this is hospital policy," he says. "We're all wearing these masks because that's the policy when anyone has a serious infection." So the patient is questioned through masks and responds to the faceless doctors gathered around him, and he is touched through thin plastic. Then we troop out of the room, strip off our masks and gloves, and, one after another, solemnly wash our hands.

Recent evidence suggests that in addition to the known routes of sexual contact and blood transfusion, AIDS may be transmitted through saliva, so it makes sense to take precautions when you do oral or rectal exams, when you draw blood, when you handle secretions. But no one thinks you can get AIDS from listening to a patient's lungs through a stethoscope or taking his pulse. In particular, you can't get AIDS by being the medical student standing in the back of the room while the resident and the interns ask the patient questions and listen to his lungs. Indeed, there is no evidence that any medical person has contracted the disease from taking care of an AIDS patient.

*   *   *

Why, then, are we all wearing masks and gloves? Sometimes we're told it's a reverse precaution—we're wearing the masks to protect the patients, who have severely compromised immune responses, from catching diseases from us. On the other hand, the patient's family and friends never wear masks, not at home and not when they visit the hospital. The gloves make no sense at all in this context. So in the end we have to face the fact that we are going through these little rituals of sanitary precaution partially because we are all terrified of this disease and are not willing to listen to anything our own dear medical profession may tell us about how it actually is or is not transmitted.

Medical people are sometimes unwilling to accept that deadly infections persist. It does not seem right to us. Throughout history there have been deadly infectious diseases, epidemics and plagues, microbes that disrupted whole civilizations, germs that killed children. Nowadays, in most of the world, this is still true. It was true when my parents were growing up in New York City; polio epidemics left empty seats in the classroom. When I was little and my parents talked about those times, they seemed very remote to me, at least as remote as Beth's death in *Little Women*. I asked my parents, "Are there still sicknesses I can catch that could kill me?" No, I was assured, because now medicines can cure all those sicknesses, and vaccines can keep you from catching them.

In recent years, for at least a certain privileged segment of the world's population, epidemics of deadly, incurable infectious diseases have not been major threats. Many diseases are dangerous to already debilitated people. Exceptionally severe infections can carry off children—or indeed anyone. But we don't live in fear of a plague.

Watching myself and the other medical people in

the hospital, I wonder if we are able to accept what has always been a central fact of the medical profession: doctors are exposed to infections. When those infections are deadly, when they are beyond the reach of vaccines and antibiotics, we are still exposed to them. When you are talking about colds and sore throats you are talking about a mild occupational hazard, an annoyance, and when you are talking about incurable diseases, then you are talking about what you might fairly call the heroism of the profession. But either way, the concept of medical professionalism does not allow for a refusal to take care of someone because you are afraid of catching a disease.

It's legitimate to feel slightly nervous drawing blood from someone with AIDS or hepatitis B or any other disease that could, theoretically, be transmitted by an accident with a needle. It's legitimate to put on a mask before examining someone with infectious tuberculosis. But when you come to the AIDS patient's door, meaning to ask him a question or two, and find a box of gloves and a box of masks and even a box of disposable surgical gowns sitting there waiting for you, and most especially when you find yourself willingly complying with the whole rigmarole and washing your hands afterward, then you have to acknowledge that something less legitimate is going on.

On the simplest level, doctors are getting spooked, responding not to a new disease but to the ancient fear of contagion, and responding with an atavistic terror that, paradoxically, uses as charms all the most modern disposable sterile safeguards. I talked with medical students who worked in other hospitals, and we all agreed that the precautions are highly erratic, varying from hospital to hospital and even within a given institution, from floor to floor, from patient to patient—

local rituals that bring comfort and security to the staff.

What do they do to the patient? Masks and gloves tend to remove what little human contact is provided by the attentions of the doctor; as an intern said of a patient with AIDS, "It's like he's in surgery, except he's awake."

I talked with a medical student who watched a good friend die of AIDS this year. The student, whose perspective lay somewhere between nondoctor and doctor, viewed the precautions partly in terms of the delicate politics of the hospital. When the policy was masks he wore a mask, specifically not to antagonize the people taking care of his friend. He also felt strongly that the precautions were the doctors' way of creating distance between themselves and the patient: "It's a way of saying, you have AIDS and I don't, you're gay and I'm not, you're going to die and I'm not, and I'm not gonna get attached to you."

This, of course, is a perennial issue for doctors, this creation of distance, and there are many methods, tangible and intangible. Every dying patient is by definition a reminder of mortality. When that patient is dying because of an infectious agent, and the mortality is, theoretically, communicable, the need for distance may transcend anything that can be established with emotional dead space. Physical barriers are needed, not because doctors think they will actually protect, but as comfortingly palpable extensions of those mental mechanisms. The fears that an epidemic like AIDS engenders may drive doctors beyond the bounds of consistency and rationalism, perhaps because they seem to come out of a more frightening past, when medicine had less power over microbes.

Taking Precautions

Danny is fourteen years old and he has diarrhea. It has been bothering him for quite a while, and it doesn't seem to be getting any better, and he has been admitted to the hospital to have it sorted out. So you're going to send off stool samples, some blood chemistries, liver function tests, and he's going to be scheduled for X rays. And since he's a hemophiliac, you're sending off blood for a screening test for HTLV-III antibodies. HTLV-III (human T-cell lymphotropic virus III, also known as LAV, for lymphadenopathy-associated virus, also known as HIV, for human immune virus) is thought to be the agent that causes AIDS, and hemophiliacs, of course, are at risk for AIDS because of frequent transfusions of blood products.

So you stamp up a bunch of lab slips, ordering the various tests this patient needs, and then you go into his room and talk for a while with Danny and his parents. He's a nice, bright kid, teasing his mother by asking if as a reward for behaving himself in the hospital he can get his hair cut in a mohawk. He has been in the hospital lots of times for bleeding problems from his hemophilia, so he's a real pro; he has his cassette player and a large stash of tapes, an enormous pile of magazines, textbooks to keep up with his schoolwork—and his father is busy hanging a life-sized poster of a hockey player on the wall.

"Well," you say cheerfully, "the vampires will be in here tomorrow morning to get your blood."

"Tell me about it," says Danny with profound scorn.

At this point a nurse comes to the door and beckons to you to go out and talk in the corridor. She saw you sending for the HTLV-III antibody test, and what she wants to know is this: do you think this patient has AIDS? Should he be on precautions—that is, should the hospital staff be warned to take special precautions when handling his blood and body fluids?

Well, you explain, the only reason we're thinking about AIDS is that he's in a high-risk group—we don't really have any other reason to suspect it. The decision of whether to put him on precautions you defer to the senior physician in charge of the case. What's bothering you is this: you don't know if anyone has yet said to Danny (or his parents), we're testing to see if you might have AIDS. You don't want to be the person to say it, but you especially don't want Danny to find PRECAUTION signs up around his bed and discover he's now being referred to by the staff as "that poor kid who has AIDS." And that's a likely turn of events if you put him on precautions.

On the other hand, of course, if you suspect a disease that might be communicated by accidents with blood and body fluids, you have a responsibility to let the staff know. But at what point? When do you mention the possibility to your patient? When do you get suspicious enough to enforce precautions?

Now it stands to reason that this patient and his parents have thought about the risk of AIDS, what with all the publicity the disease has gotten. They know hemophiliacs are considered a high-risk group, surely, and probably AIDS flickers across their minds with any new illness. But still, that doesn't mean they've faced up to the possibility that Danny's diarrhea could be the first manifestation of a fatal illness. Do they really need you to march in and say, of course we're checking you out for AIDS, because that conceivably could explain your symptoms? Wouldn't it be kinder to wait till there are some test results? Suppose you find an explanation for the symptoms that has nothing to do with immune deficiency—an intestinal parasite like *Giardia,* for example, that he might have picked up on his camping trip last summer if he drank from streams contaminated by infected beavers (you would love to be able to offer this mildly comical etiology to Danny and his parents, this benign, curable condition). If another explanation is in fact going to turn up, why give them all days of anxiety by letting them think you suspect it's AIDS?

Ideally, you would know your patient well, you would have a relationship based on trust and confidence, an understanding of the particular emotional variables involved, and ample time for discussion. You would be able to sit down and explain carefully what the various possibilities are, even the worst ones, offering rationales and reassurance. And sometimes you can. But often the patient is someone you don't know at all, and time is limited. You have to pick your words carefully.

There are certain words that almost nobody wants to hear. Up until recently, "cancer" was the most deadly, the word not to be mentioned in front of a patient. Not until it was a sure and certain diagnosis— and even then many doctors preferred to use other terms, like "melanoma" or "malignant polyps," more specific and less terrifying, regardless of the actual prognosis. In other times or other places, other words have conveyed that sudden shocking horror—"tuberculosis," "leprosy," words that couldn't be mentioned as casual possibilities because they would come to dominate all others in the patient's mind, because the suggestion might be taken as confirmation of that patient's worst and most tightly repressed fears.

And that's one of the problems with this approach: frequently the word you're avoiding is also the word that keeps resounding loudly in your patient's brain—I don't have cancer, do I? You don't think this is AIDS? And it's a very tricky thing to judge when a particular patient needs to hear you discuss the worst-case possibility and when a patient would rather not hear about it unless you have definite news.

After all, we run a lot of tests on a lot of patients —that's what hospitals do. And frequently tests are run just for completeness (or occasionally for compulsive completeness, as in, this patient was tested for a large number of completely unlikely syndromes because his doctor is a total anal-compulsive). Doctors say to each other, let's just rule out this, that, and the other thing. So you don't necessarily go in and give the patient a list of all the arcane things you're ruling out, a nice big set of terrible and highly unlikely diseases that your poor patient may never even have heard of: well, here are some new things to worry about. No, you obviously don't do that.

On the other hand, when there's a serious possibility you think needs to be mentioned, you want to be sure it's done carefully. You don't want a new doctor (or medical student) the patient has never seen before to come barging into the room and say loudly to a resident, is this the guy who has cancer? And you don't want newly hung PRECAUTION signs to communicate your message.

Some patients spare you this tangle of decisions. They let you know right away what they're worried about. In other instances, you may have to guess at the source of a patient's anxiety that has no relation to reality. For example, an adolescent who comes into your emergency room with pain in his chest may be absolutely certain he's having a heart attack, while that possibility may be so low on your list that you don't even think to mention it. It takes a certain amount of imagination to provide the right kind of reassurance.

What are you going to do about Danny? Are you going to go into his room, sit his parents down in chairs next to his bed, and begin talking about AIDS? Wouldn't you rather wait until the HTLV-III antibody test comes back? But here's the thing—this test can't actually be used to diagnose AIDS. All it shows is that someone has been exposed to the virus and has developed antibodies to it. It doesn't mean that the virus is still present or that the patient will develop the disease. And because of their exposure to blood products, a great many hemophiliacs will in fact have positive tests, so what are you going to tell him if the test is positive?

And for that matter, as long as we're talking about sticky issues of this kind, what about the patient who has no symptoms that make you suspect AIDS, but is in the hospital for another reason (injured hand got infected, flare-up of old ulcers) and gets an HTLV-III test sent off just because he happens to be in a high-risk group for AIDS and some doctor is curious? Is this patient's privacy being violated? Does he have the right to know that the test is being sent? And if it comes back positive, which isn't diagnostic of anything, what then? Will he suddenly find himself put on precautions?

In the end, it comes down to this: doctors don't usually consider it part of good care to explain all the details of their thinking to their patients. Instead they say, we're running some tests to see if we can locate the problem, we're checking some cultures to see if you have an infection, we're going to take a look inside your digestive tract to see if everything's okay. It isn't considered necessary for the doctor to let the patient in on every single possibility, to describe every single blood test and the ramifications of a hypothetical positive or negative. And so doctors take refuge behind this general rule when it comes to the problem of terrifying words, deadly diagnoses. And there's a needle-fine line that good doctors must walk, a desperately sensitive balance to preserve, which consists of understanding for each individual patient: does this person need to hear me discuss the possibility or need not to hear it? The patient's needs have to be reflected back off the doctor's perceptions, and the skill of those perceptions will determine whether the doctor's words bring catharsis, comfort, or catastrophe.

You want to know what happened to Danny, don't you? You want an answer, and there is no clear answer. His HTLV-III antibody test came back positive and he was in fact placed on precautions. Meanwhile, no *Giardia* was found, but his doctor decided to try him on a course of antiparasite medication—and his diarrhea did abate. A gastroenterologist who examined him thought he might have inflammatory bowel disease, but was unable to say for sure. So he goes home without a definite answer, to wait and see what happens, and to phrase his worries to himself in whatever words he chooses.

The preceding two essays are somewhat out of date. When I was a third-year medical student, AIDS was still a comparatively unusual diagnosis in the hospitals where I worked. Since then, it has become far more common, and it is now dealt with routinely by hospital staff. The extreme precautions described in "AIDS" are rarely observed. The HTLV-III antibody test discussed in "Taking Precautions" cannot be done without the patient's permission (or the patient's parent's permission). These essays describe aspects of the medical profession's early attempts to deal with the AIDS epidemic. Now we are all much more experienced, and we face a new set of problems—which is another story.

Dying

Perhaps you remember how Beth dies in *Little Women*. Knowing she is dying, she offers words of wisdom and comfort to her sorrowing sister Jo, telling her, "You must take my place, Jo, and be everything to Father and Mother when I'm gone. They will turn to you, don't fail them; and if it's hard to work alone, remember that I don't forget you, and that you'll be happier in doing that than writing splendid books or seeing all the world; for love is the only thing that we can carry with us when we go, and it makes the end so easy."

And Jo is helped and comforted by these words. " 'I'll try, Beth,' and there and then Jo renounced her old ambition, pledged herself to a new and better one, acknowledging the poverty of other desires, and feeling the blessed solace of a belief in the immortality of love.' "

Beth gets the death scene she deserves, of course, peaceful and gentle, in her mother's arms, and "the spring sunshine streamed in like a benediction over the placid face upon the pillow—a face so full of painless peace that those who loved it best smiled through their tears, and thanked God that Beth was well at last."

Now, I have cried over Beth's death a good many times in my life. She is by no means my favorite character in the book, of course, what with her steady, gentle goodness, honesty, and piety, but I think I never quite got over the feeling that as an invalid, as a girl with a fatal illness, she is model. That is the right way to sicken, the right way to die. Consider, for example, the way she gets sick in the first place—by going to bring comfort to a poor miserable family of immigrants whose child promptly dies in Beth's lap, passing on to her the scarlet fever from which she apparently never fully recovers. Yes, absolutely, a person who is going to get sick and die had better behave like a saint. I think I knew always, through my tears, that I didn't have it in me.

I thought of Beth March one day during my first year of medical school. As part of the very earliest introduction to the hospital, to clinical medicine, a doctor had arranged a visit with a patient. Another student and I were to meet with this boy, who had agreed to talk to us about his illness, muscular dystrophy, a genetic disorder that allows normal intellectual development but involves progressive physical debilitation. To quote the information booklet we give out to patients, "improved medical care is increasing the lifespan . . . but rarely beyond early adulthood."

The patient was a small, thin twelve-year-old boy. He looked up as we came into the room, and called out to us, "So, you're the people who want to hear me talk about what it feels like to be dying and all that jazz." And talk to us he did: he spoke at length about the incompetence of some of the doctors who had treated him, about how an intern had once tried to prescribe for him a medicine that was dangerous for people with his disease, how he had been forced to go over the intern's head and call in a senior doctor who had confirmed that he was right and the intern wrong. He told us about other people with muscular dystrophy he had known who were now dead, and explained

to us why each of them had done something or other
to make death inevitable, concluding each time, "I'm
sure not gonna do that."

The phone next to his bed rang and he snatched up
the receiver: "Herman's Mortuary, you stab 'em, we
slab 'em."

A little while later, his mother came in and told us
he was doing very well, that she hoped he'd be leaving
soon. The child cackled, "Well, one way or another
I'll be leaving soon, right, Ma? It's either leave in a
car or leave in a box!" His mother looked exasper-
ated, in the manner of mothers of twelve-year-old
boys who are acting up in front of company. We, the
company, did not meet her eyes.

After we left his hospital room, we exchanged a few
tentative sentences about how sad it was, how bright
he seemed, how hard it must be for his family. Then,
rather in a rush, the other medical student said, "I
don't know if I could deal with having a patient like
that. Lecturing like that about what's wrong with the
doctors? And making those jokes all the time?" And
the doctor nodded, looking sad, and I nodded too,
agreeing.

And there I was, thinking about Beth March, and
also thinking, for the first time in my whole life, that if
I were dying, what I would probably be like was that
boy we had just talked to. Obnoxious, wise-ass, trying
to be funny, searching for a good line at the expense
of my doctor, or my mother, always alert for incompetence in the people taking care of me. Nothing like
Beth. No inspiration for those I would be leaving
behind. No wisdom, no comfort, no storybook bravery. And with that thought came a shock of recognition, as if I had truly seen myself on my deathbed.

People who are sick do not necessarily behave well.
Certainly they do not even come close to the Holly-
wood ideal, the disease that kills off Ali MacGraw

without damaging her looks or her spunk. People who are sick get pugnacious, or uncooperative, or desperately cranky. They yell at their relatives, complain about their nurses, accuse their doctors of incompetence. And somehow, through it all, I think many of us who take care of sick people preserve this idea that they have some responsibility to behave in an exemplary style. We expect courage, quiet trust (in us, of course), gentle uncomplaining fortitude. And when we get it, as sometimes happens, we tend to be pleased; those people make good patients. They're grateful for the care they get, they don't yell too loudly when you stick needles into them, they manage a smile in the morning when you wake them up on rounds. They are truly and profoundly admirable.

But what do you do on morning rounds when the man in the bed looks up at the resident and says, "Doctor, I've been here for two weeks and you tell me you still don't know what's wrong with me. I'm gonna die here, and you'll be standing there with a stupid expression on your face, wondering what was the matter. I'm paying through the nose for this, and you're gonna let me die!"

Or what about a patient who clings to your hand and says, over and over, "I don't want to die, please promise you won't let me die."

And when you think about it, either of those responses makes more sense than gentle good behavior. Still, doctors frequently don't know quite how to cope. I remember a four-year-old boy who was dying; he screamed and carried on and attacked any doctor who came near him. So we asked a child psychiatrist to come by and see him, and the child psychiatrist reported back to us that he was terrified of dying. Pause. "Actually, that's quite appropriate under the circumstances," the psychiatrist told us, gently.

What else is appropriate under the circumstances?

Is it appropriate to resent the people who will be left behind to continue living? Is it appropriate to wish that someone else would die instead of you? Is it appropriate to pick out a person or two in particular? Or is it just appropriate to lie in bed all day and quake with fear? Is it appropriate to be grateful for the medical care you get, even if it is not going to save your life, or is it more appropriate to hate your doctors and your nurses for their impending failure? What do the circumstances demand?

The circumstances are impossible. Most people do not want to die, do not see any reason why they should be dying and the world moving on steadily without them. In fact, it is remarkable that people behave as well as they do. And all the obvious truths apply: it sometimes helps to be religious, it is sometimes easier to face dying if you're tired out after a long and miserable illness. But for people facing death with neither serenity nor acceptance, doctors may not have much to offer.

Of course, doctors do not face the death of a patient with either serenity or acceptance. Many complaints have been entered about the unwillingness of the medical profession to allow inevitable death without frantic invasive interventions. The doctor would ideally walk a careful line, fighting as long as fighting is worthwhile, withdrawing from the battle when it is clearly futile. But when you train people to think in terms of doing everything that can be done, approaching illness aggressively and energetically, well, it gets to be very hard for them to turn off those attitudes even when all their aggression and energy are clearly doomed to failure. And so doctors find themselves in the same bind as patients, and unable to accept death gracefully, they may make a patient's dying hideous with medical invasions.

This, however, is not seen as the patient's job. The

patient's role is to accept what is done by the doctors, but when the doctors fail, to accept that failure with good grace and saintly demeanor. One imagines Beth March's doctors, off in the next room, coming up with one new possible treatment after another, even though her illness, Terminal Too-Good-to-Live Disease, has never, in the whole history of literature, successfully been cured. Think of Little Eva, in *Uncle Tom's Cabin*. Think of Dora, in *David Copperfield*.

A good patient, then, is a patient who accepts the decisions of more powerful forces, most notably the doctors, but also the decisions of fate. The good patient is resigned, but also willing to allow the medical battle to continue as long as the doctors feel it to be necessary, and in addition, the good patient is grateful for that battle, no matter how painful or debilitating or fruitless it may prove.

And there just aren't all that many good patients around. Probably we would all like to imagine ourselves facing death well. In fact, our expectations of how very ill patients should behave may have less to do with the clichés of literature than with our fantasies of how we would face our own ends. In some way it seems to resolve the whole issue of human mortality if you imagine for yourself a sickbed fraught with wisdom, serenity, the glad consciousness of a life well lived, and a proud and heroic courage in the face of the unknowable. Yes indeed. And doctors need to "resolve" human mortality somehow or other; they have to face too much of it to leave it nagging at them. It is not in any way comforting to picture a death that involves extended whining, or frequent eruptions of anger and frustration. So you work in the hospital a lot, you sometimes find yourself imagining how you would act in those extreme situations, and I'm afraid that my vision of myself has come to include more than a little whining. I end up hoping that I would have as much courage as that twelve-year-old boy, courage manifested not in wise comforting speeches or saintly joy in the inevitable, but in the maintenance of spirit and individuality in impossible circumstances. Not to mention humor, of whatever kind.

As we stood in his hospital room, after a while we ran out of questions, too intimidated by the sadness of the situation to come up with any intelligent conversation. So the patient lectured us for a while about his disease.

The other medical student thought of a question. "Are you interested in medicine?" she asked.

"Well," he said, "not by choice."

Curing

Now, when I say, go watch some small children playing doctor, I m not telling you to interfere in matters that deserve strict privacy. Not that kind of playing doctor. I mean, go watch some little kids playing the kind of doctor that involves a little plastic stethoscope, a teeny-weeny blood pressure cuff, and a needleless hypodermic—one of those sets parents give to children for reasons that don't really bear close examination. Watch the way the game is played. Someone gets sick, comes to the "doctor." Intent listening with the stethoscope, creative use of the blood pressure cuff, any other diagnostic procedures that come to mind—I've seen impressive use of the reflex hammer, for example. And then the diagnosis is made, and therapy is instituted immediately: an injection, maybe a red-hot or an M&M, and, in really critical cases, a Band-Aid. And the patient is cured. All better.

And to tell the truth, that paradigm is not so very different from the kind of medicine I grew up watching on television, and since this was my main source of information about doctors and what they do, I think it's more or less what I expected to do with my life. A man gets sick. You examine him. You find out what's wrong. You cure him. I sort of imagined an endless cabinet of medicines, each marked with the name of a specific sickness.

So here we are on morning rounds in the hospital,

with real stethoscopes draped round our necks. And in this room is your basic adult medicine elective admission, a CAD for cath and probably CABG (pronounced "cabbage")—a patient with coronary artery disease, here for cardiac catheterization and probably a coronary artery bypass graft operation (got that? now say "CAD-for-cath-and-CABG" ten times fast). And in the next room is a patient with inflammatory bowel disease. And next is a room with two chronic lungers, or COPDers (for "chronic obstructive pulmonary disease"), one of whom may have lung cancer; the other just has bad shortness of breath. And next is an old woman from a nursing home with FTT—failure to thrive (she keeps losing weight and no one can find a reason).

I promise you, I'm not stacking the deck. This is a very common set of patients. But guess what? We can't cure any of them. Coronary artery bypass surgery is a procedure people swear by, but its efficacy in prolonging life is disputed. Though it may make the patient more comfortable, it certainly doesn't reverse the blood vessel disease. Inflammatory bowel disease is treated with symptomatic relief, with drugs that sometimes heal the bowel but have serious side effects, and if those fail, by surgical removal of parts of the bowel, which sometimes leaves the patient with a colostomy. And then, with any luck, the parts of the bowel left don't develop the disease. Chronic lung disease has no treatment; you try to get the patient to stop smoking, and you give medicines that make breathing easier, but you can't reverse the damage to the lungs. Failure to thrive—well, if you could find a cause, you might be able to cure it, but an awful lot of failure to thrive is idiopathic—which is jargon for "of no known cause."

I don't mean to be overly depressing. There's a lot of hope that the hospital may be able to offer these patients, hope for improved quality of life, longer life—but not cure. Get that word right out of your mind. Stroke your stethoscope, finger your reflex hammer, and adjust to reality.

And yet many people come into emergency rooms expecting that the doctors are going to be able to cure what ails them. And the really remakable thing is that even well into their careers, doctors too sometimes find themselves thinking along those lines. There are certain illnesses for which the medical response actually does fit that paradigm, and when you learn about them, they tell you, "And this one really makes you feel like a doctor."

Allergic skin reactions, for example. Someone comes in miserable after a bee sting, and you give a little epinephrine and the problem goes away in a matter of seconds. Severe diarrhea and dehydration—the child comes in lying limp, looks dead. Hook up an IV, give some fluid fast, and the kid jumps off the stretcher, smiling; the parents think you're God. Some infectious diseases—gonorrhea, for example, or most kinds of bacterial pneumonia—can also be treated.

Here are some things that come into the emergency room and can't be cured. A few you know—the common cold, most sore throats. Herpes. Also most heart disease, most lung disease. In other words, big things and little things. So how does the medical profession deal with this fact of life? How does this figure in the teaching of medical students?

When you study pathophysiology, when you learn the diseases of the various organ systems, you learn the pathology, epidemiology, clinical course, and complications for each disease, and you also learn the therapy and the prognosis. So, disease by disease, you come to understand that therapeutic possibilities vary tremendously. You get used to looking for such euphemisms as "therapy—supportive" (keep the patient nourished, breathing, and wait for the disease to get either better or worse). Then there's "therapy—alleviation of symptoms" or "therapy—comfort measures." One of the most famous medical textbooks, Harrison's *Principles of Internal Medicine* (a 2,212-page work that most of us have committed to memory) tries on page 3 to explain what doctors can do when they have no effective therapy to offer: "in those cases which do not lend themselves to easy solutions or for which no effective treatment is available, a feeling on the part of the patient that the physician is doing all that is possible is one of the most important therapeutic measures that can be provided."

And in fact this sometimes leads to doctors going overboard, trying one test after another, one procedure after another, just to demonstrate to the patient and the patient's family that an effort is being made, precisely because the doctors don't really believe in a cure.

There's also a tendency to search hopefully for a treatable disease, and a deep fear of missing such a disease. You'll go down a list of possible causes for some symptom or other, and then your teacher will say forcefully, now *this* one is important, because this one we can treat. There are so many things you can find but not treat; don't miss the ones you can treat.

But basically, when you come right down to it, it's frustrating for a lot of people. It's frustrating to want to cure, to carry with you the expectation that somehow you *should* be able to cure, and then not be able to cure. It can make you dislike particular diseases, and even particular patients. Doctors are notoriously bad with dying patients, those emblems of medical failure, and sometimes the patient who isn't actually dying, but who's sick with some chronic and incurable disease, can present the same kind of unpleasant prospect.

Maybe the whole model of curing disease is wrong. Maybe it's simply unrealistic to think in those terms. Medicine has been taken to task often enough in recent years for ignoring preventive care and what have come to be called life-style issues. Maybe we should be concentrating on diet and exercise, stress reduction. Maybe we need, as well, to come to terms with the process of aging, to get rid of this idea that all the changes in the body tissues should ideally be reversible. Maybe we need to revise the concept of disease states to take greater account of chronic conditions. All this would mean rethinking the doctor's role.

Because the doctor's role, of course, is to cure. In defiance of the facts that most doctors face every day, the role is still, somehow, to cure. It's the model, the ideal.

So this eighteen-year-old kid comes into the hospital with a story of nausea, vomiting, followed by some sleepiness, general grogginess. And it turns out that what's wrong with him is diabetic ketoacidosis, an acute complication of diabetes. This guy never knew he had diabetes, mind you, and now he finds himself in the hospital the next morning and a doctor is trying to explain something to him. He's going to need to take insulin from now on, watch what he eats and drinks, see a doctor regularly.

So the patient asks the obvious question: you mean there isn't any cure?

Well, says the doctor, we can control it very well now. Not adding, since there's no need to drop all the bad news at once, that there are a number of very serious long-term complications of diabetes that this young man may eventually have to worry about. And that the evidence everyone hoped to find, the evidence that close control of blood sugar levels will help prevent some of these complications—well, that evidence has been ambiguous.

Now here's someone who has a disease but who can go on living his life; his life isn't over, or even destroyed. He's lucky to be alive now, rather than seventy years ago, because medical science can do much more for him now. And yet it's still very limited. In the end, his doctor has to sigh and think of Harrison again, page 678 this time (see, I did get past page 3), the chapter on diabetes: "Acceptance of the fact that a person has a chronic disease which requires a complete change in life-style is always difficult. This is particularly true in the case of diabetes since patients generally are aware that they are vulnerable to late complications and that statistically their life expectancy is shortened."

When I started my clerkship in internal medicine, the resident who was supervising my team said to me, "Well, we don't cure anybody, but we have a lot of fun." He was joking, maybe a little desperately, but he was also telling at least some of the truth. And even though you learn individually, disease by disease, about the limitations of medicine, somehow the overall message is to cure. And during your training you have to come to terms, all by yourself, with the reality that most of what you do has little to do with curing. Sometimes you make people better. Often they get better by themselves. Sometimes you make them more comfortable while they get sicker. Sometimes you make them more miserable while they get sicker. Maybe what we need is an increased level of respect both for the patient's own ability to get better and for the power of disease. Maybe we need to revise our role so that we're more comfortable being a little more passive. I don't know; I'm not really ready to make that adjustment (instead, I'm going into pediatrics, where more of the patients get better because more of the patients were healthy to begin with).

My friend Mitch, a fellow medical student, summed it up in TV voice-over tones: "Another day in the hospital, subjecting the sick to painful and useless invasive procedures, and curing the healthy."

Assess and Advise

The newborn intensive care unit is well lit, because an intensive care unit has to be well lit; the nurses and doctors have to be able to read the gauges, graphs, and monitors attached to each patient, they have to be able to check for small changes in the patient's coloring or breathing pattern. It's accepted that the stress of noise or overly harsh lighting can be dangerous to newborns, and so every effort is made to keep such stress to a minimum. Still, intensive care means close monitoring, in all possible respects, and close monitoring demands good lighting. The machines hum and gently beep, and the nurses and doctors move about dressed in green cotton scrub suits, worn in an attempt to keep the room a little freer from contamination by outside microbes. But the bodies of the patients are so tiny; the biggest are no bigger than a normal newborn, seven or eight pounds, and the smallest . . . the smallest nowadays can weigh about a pound. There's really no margin for error with these patients, and everything from the temperature of the air around them (regulated by individual heaters and lights) to the amounts of fluid running through intravenous lines into their minute veins has to be perfectly controlled.

I'm a medical student spending a month on the neurology service; we've been called over to evaluate a newborn baby. Walking into the intensive care unit, we pass double bulletin boards covered with snapshots of "graduates," healthy children shown at their second or third birthday parties, even a couple of before-and-after combinations, in which the before is a pitifully tiny premature infant, tubes running in and out of all possible apertures, and the after is a chunky little bruiser of a toddler, ready to take over the world.

But the baby we've been called to see isn't premature. He's a full-term infant, transported in from another hospital, with a very incomplete story about what happened during his birth. Evidently, the doctor who delivered him thinks there was a severe "birth accident"—the baby was deprived of oxygen for a prolonged period because the umbilical cord was wrapped around his neck. The baby didn't start breathing after he was born, and several unsuccessful attempts were made to resuscitate him; finally they managed to get a breathing tube down his throat, and they transferred him to this big teaching hospital, and here he lies, connected to a ventilator.

The neurologists have been asked to "assess this compromised newborn's neurological status, and advise as to likely neurological prognosis." In other words, the doctors caring for this baby want an opinion about how badly damaged he is. In fact, they believe he's very badly damaged, and one of the things they're already thinking about is, are we going to need to turn off the respirator? Is this baby "brain dead"?

I watch a neurology fellow and a senior neurologist patiently going over the baby. Compared to some of the tiny bodies around him, he looks large and plump and healthy—or as healthy as you can look when attached to a ventilator, several intravenous lines, and all the rest of it. The neurologists lift the baby and pull on his limbs, checking for muscle tone. They shine lights in his eyes to see if his pupils change size. They tap him with a hammer, checking for reflexes, even pinch him to see if he responds to pain. Finally they ask for some ice water and drizzle a little into one ear to see if the baby's eyes move to one side or the other in response to this stimulus.

The concept of brain death has been both difficult and necessary for some time now. You can often keep a body going for quite a while after the brain has essentially quit. There have been court cases fought by families wanting to turn off respirators, and at least for extreme cases, most medical centers now observe certain guidelines for defining brain death. These usually involve such criteria as the absence of reflexes and the presence of a flat EEG (electroencephalograms indicate brain activity) and aren't actually very controversial in themselves. By the time a patient fulfills such stringent requirements, turning off a respirator is often the only possible action. The problem, of course, comes with all those who don't exactly fit the criteria, who show a tiny bit of activity on the EEG, or a single paradoxical reflex. For such people, also neurologically devastated beyond any hope of recovery, also "brain dead" by any but the most niggling criteria, the decision has to be made carefully and with respect, by the family and the doctors together. And all this, though it smacks of sensationalism and scandal, and interminable theoretical discussions about the ethics of such decision making, is also a very basic taken-for-granted fact of hospital life. The decision to turn off a respirator is one that's made all the time in a big hospital, in an intensive care unit. It's never made casually, not made unilaterally by doctors, not made without warning—but it's a decision that's faced, and made, all the time.

With a newborn baby, things get a little more complex, both for the doctors trying to assess the medical prognosis and for the family. As with an adult, an infant who's at the far end of the spectrum, who obviously meets all possible criteria for brain death, presents a less difficult medical problem; as I heard one doctor say, the prognosis is nonexistent. But a baby can be severely damaged and still display some evidence that a small part of the brain has been spared, that the most rigorous definition doesn't apply. And with a newborn, in these slightly unclear cases, the decision is probably even more agonizing than it is for an adult. After all, miracles somehow seem more within reach when you're dealing with children, and in fact, the regenerative powers of the very young can seem downright miraculous. Everyone in pediatrics has heard about cases, or seen cases, where children gained back much more function than had been predicted, where parental love and the normal biological urge to grow and be healthy somehow overcame seemingly impossible handicaps. Still, there are limits, and I'm talking about the cases that lie way out beyond those limits. And even so, with an infant, because an infant is by definition the beginning of things, there's a tremendous urge to hope.

The brightest spots in the newborn intensive care units are the colored signs on the little beds (and incubators): "I'm a girl!" "My name is Albert!" Also, there are stuffed animals tucked along the edges of some of the beds, or snapshots of parents taped to the Plexiglas crib walls. These determinedly cheerful bits of personal detail remind everyone that each miniature specimen, silent beneath its electric warmer, fed through a tube, breathing by means of a machine, is infinitely important to one particular family. In this bed is more than the sum total of a set of very difficult medical problems and maintenance equations; in this bed is a baby girl, whose parents have named her Rachel, and at home, waiting for her, they have a crib, and a bunch of tiny sleepers, and a herd of stuffed animals donated by grandparents and aunts and uncles. And they want her to come home to them, and learn to sit, and eat from a spoon, and walk and talk, and they come in every day and stare down at her, and they taped their photo to the IV pole so the photo looks down on her when they aren't there.

Now, what are the doctors going to tell the parents of that new little boy? Are they going to tell them, start hoping, start coming in to visit, bring in a teddy bear, whisper his name to him? Or are they going to tell them, it's time to mourn; what we have here is essentially a stillbirth. After all, the tragedy of a stillbirth is different from the tragedy of a living baby dying. And it would be unkind to leave the parents stranded during a period of confusion; if a painful decision has to be made it is better to make it sooner than later. To leave the parents wondering, is there in fact a baby to root for, is a harsh and terrible thing to do, and at times it's necessary; if in doubt, you have to wait and see.

And while you wait and see, heroism may be made manifest as the parents learn to love and cherish the tiny body kept alive by the ventilator, and with all the love, the decision grows more difficult—which is, of course, appropriate.

We stand there in the newborn intensive care unit. The baby is going to be somewhere close to the terrible end of the spectrum. But his EEG isn't actually flat, and when ice water is poured into his ear, his eyes seem to deviate a little, though it isn't easy to tell. He's going to have a more precise test to evaluate this response, and another EEG. To be honest, all the doctors standing around this little bed are basically in agreement: they don't think this baby stands a chance. They think his brain has been completely devastated, and there is no hope of recovery. The tests they're scheduling—and they've now put together a substantial list—are to reassure themselves that they're not making a mistake, to enable them to reassure the baby's parents that they've checked and double-checked. In fact, the doctors aren't yet saying, even to each other, that this respirator is going to have to be turned off. They're not absolutely ready to stop hoping, even though they think that the most that could possibly be hoped for would still be pretty terrible—that is, a child who would live, but would be very severely damaged.

There are no words, really, for the tragedy of this small perfect body without a functioning brain. There are not even the conventional words of sympathy you offer to parents—how lucky you are to have known this child, to have had your lives enriched by this child. What the parents will mourn is the loss of hopes and plans and fond expectations. They will find that as well as the death of their child, they must mourn the death of dreams, and all because that child, though intact in body, has lost the organ where dreams are made.

It isn't easy to rule and advise in such circumstances. You do your best, bring as much expertise, as many potentially useful tests as you think are necessary. You try to give this decision the weight it deserves, understanding that it deserves, in fact, the weight of a lifetime.

DNR

"So, what are the issues on this patient?" asked the resident, after I had finished my presentation.

I was ready for this. "Her issues are, one, her congestive heart failure, two, her renal failure—"

The resident interrupted me. "What's her most important issue?"

Had I missed something? I backtracked hastily. "Well, of course, I see what you mean, her most important issue really isn't her heart failure, it's her pneumonia, I should have put that first—"

"Wrong," said the resident. "Her most important issue is status. We need to get a status on her today."

Status means, is this patient DNR or not? DNR, which stands for "do not resuscitate," means no heroic measures in the event that the patient seems about to die. If the breathing stops, no artificial ventilator. If the heart stops, no pounding on the chest, no electric shocks. And no code. When the non-DNR patient looks about to die, you call a code, an emergency announcement is broadcast throughout the hospital, and everyone who can comes to help. With the DNR patient, there is no code.

Ideally, status is the patient's own decision. If the patient is not mentally intact, the decision may be made by the family. Obviously, it is a tremendously touchy subject to negotiate with a family; people may feel terribly guilty about agreeing to let a parent or

sibling be made DNR. People choose to be made
DNR, understanding for example that their medical
condition is such that once on a mechanical ventilator,
they are unlikely ever to come off it. They choose to
be DNR because they feel that because of age, or
severity of sickness, or level of pain, if death should
come they would like it to come peacefully. No room
crowded with doctors and nurses and medical students
and technicians. No technological "miracles" bringing
them back from the dead. As one patient said, "If you
could cure what ails me, that would be a miracle worth
having. Bringing me back so I can die of this same
thing a little way down the line, that isn't even a
favor."

In principle, then, DNR is a very good thing. It
allows patients, or at least those who love them best,
to make a very important decision. People don't get to
choose the circumstances of their deaths, by and large.
The hospital, as has often been pointed out, is not
really a very good place to die, far from familiar
surroundings, far from the small and all-important comforts of home. In that setting, the question of whether
or not the patient wishes to be DNR restores some
measure of dignity and authority.

Here is a joke a friend told me, another medical
student. It is a joke which was current in the hospital
where he was working, a joke told by doctors about
the things we do to dying patients and the difficulty of
avoiding them.

Three explorers are captured by an extremely hostile tribe and are tied to stakes. The chieftain ap-
proaches and offers the first explorer a choice, death
or *chi-chi*. The crowd of tribespeople is screaming,
"Chi-chi! Chi-chi!" The first explorer, thinking anything is better than death, chooses *chi-chi*. He is un-
tied, thrown down on a table, stripped naked, every

orifice is violated, tubes are stuck into his body, he is cut with knives, and then he is killed. The second explorer is offered the same choice, chooses *chi-chi,* and is treated exactly like the first. The third explorer is asked, "Death or *chi-chi?*" "*Chi-chi!*" screams the crowd. The explorer chooses death. "Death?" says the chieftain. "Nobody ever chose death before. . . . Okay, death! But first—*chi-chi!*"

Like most people who work in hospitals, I believe that the major danger is still too much intervention, not too little. DNR status is not a sinister trap which is sprung on the unwary; it is intended as an honest attempt to save sick people from useless agonies. And yet, as with so much else in the hospital, the question of status is affected by the field of pressure surrounding the doctors.

"I know what you guys like, you like people to be DNR, the more the better," I heard a senior doctor tell a group of interns and residents, trying to get a rise out of them. "It means less trouble for you at night if something happens."

Well, no, that isn't really true. It's not a question of avoiding trouble, it's just that the intern, left alone at night in charge of very sick patients, may be terrified of not being able to handle an emergency, and may be relieved if some of the sickest people are DNR. It's a natural relief; if the worst happens, the intern is not responsible for keeping the patient alive. Doctors can get very annoyed with patients or families who insist on refusing the DNR status in the face of medical advice; some of the annoyance may be on the patient's own behalf, but much of it stems from the knowledge that they, the doctors, may have to spend time and effort and hospital resources to resuscitate a patient whom they have decided is essentially beyond medical aid. And that annoyance, which is perfectly justifiable on any number of grounds, may lead doctors to pressure patients and families a little, or at least to present the decision in less than balanced terms.

The other problem with DNR, of course, is that no one is exactly sure what it means. That is, everyone knows it means no code, no heroic measures at the moment of death. But what about before? Do you perform surgery on a patient who is DNR? Do you do painful investigative procedures? Theoretically, the DNR status should not affect any of these other decisions, but in fact it's sometimes taken to indicate a general desire on the part of the patient or family for minimal intervention. That may indeed be what the patient wants, but it is also true that sometimes when a patient is made DNR, the doctor's attitude changes. Because the patient has decided against the ultimate in medical aggressiveness, some doctors may become less aggressive in other ways as well. It is almost as if, for certain doctors, once a patient has been officially ruled beyond the reach of medical heroism, that patient ceases to exist as a medical problem.

"I don't make my patients DNR if I expect them to leave the hospital alive," said that same senior doctor, taking an extreme position. Most doctors would argue that there are different kinds of DNR. There is the person who stands a good chance of walking out of the hospital, but who wants to die peacefully if his heart stops. And then there is the person who will be dead in a matter of days and is in constant pain. In the one case you may want to proceed with all sorts of aggressive therapies, and in the other you may even stop taking the patient's temperature, because you don't want to know if an infection develops.

But it is not always clear that the patient, in agreeing to be DNR, understands where on that spectrum his doctor considers him to be. And so it does happen that a family reluctantly allows a dying parent to be made DNR, expecting it to be interpreted in its strictest sense, and the doctors use it as a license for a general pull-back. And it also happens, and probably more frequently, that as in the *chi-chi* joke a patient chooses to be DNR, hoping to die quickly and peacefully, and still receives every possible unwanted medical attention, simply because the doctor's reflexes are too strong. Such patients get tested regularly for problems that cannot be corrected or if temporarily corrected only prolong death agonies they wish to shorten.

When the resident said, "Her most important issue is status," what he meant was, if she starts to die tonight, can I let her? The responsibilities weighing on the doctors, the genuine humanitarian concerns, and the strong impulses to act aggressively are not easy to sort out. The patient makes a choice. The doctor interprets the choice. Patient and doctor are locked together in a situation that marks the end of life for one, the height of professional complexity for the other. Either they will understand each other or they will not, and the level of understanding they achieve will determine the real meaning of the patient's chosen status and, in another sense, the doctor's status as well.

PUTTING IT TOGETHER

[Queen Victoria to Sir Robert Peel]
7th September 1841

The Queen wishes that Sir Robert Peel would mention to Lord De la Warr that he should be very particular in always naming to the Queen any appointment he wishes to make in his department, and always to take her pleasure upon an appointment before he settles on them; this is a point upon which the Queen has always laid great stress. This applies in great measure to the appointment of Physicians and Chaplains, which used to be very badly managed formerly, and who were appointed in a very careless manner; but since the Queen's accession the Physicians and Chaplains have been appointed only for merit and abilities, by the Queen herself, which the Queen is certain Sir Robert Peel will at once see is a far better way, and one which must be of use in every way.

Queen Victoria's Early Letters

A MEDICAL EDUCATION IS NOT, of course, an end in itself. It is meant to prepare you for what comes next, and I am aware that as I write this, at the end of my four years of medical school, my perspective has by no means stopped changing. The next few years will involve transitions as great or greater; I will have to go from being a student to being a doctor, and then a doctor who supervises other doctors. I cannot begin to guess how I will think and feel at the end of my residency, because I frankly cannot yet imagine myself with that level of competence.

Still, what I want to do in this last section is to look ahead, to put together the fund of pathophysiological knowledge I have acquired, the experience of clinical clerkship, the overwhelming ethical and personal issues to be resolved, and also what I have seen of the training of interns and residents. In the long piece that follows, I have tried to show how the pressures of time and weariness and personality can act on medical students and young doctors in the hospital; to give some impression of what this world I have come to know can be like. I have also included a piece about finishing fourth year, coming to terms, somehow, with the next step. Unbelievably, disbelievingly, eagerly, but also with tremendous trepidation, I am going to become a doctor.

The essay that follows is not specifically, or not

explicitly, about me. The medical student is described in the third person, and both the patients and the doctors are composite figures, though all the incidents described really happened. Perhaps in my attempt to convey the hospital I have reverted to the form of writing that I have loved best all my life, and borrowed some methods from the short story. Although it is in fact not fiction, I would like this article to do for the nondoctor what some fiction does for me, to conjure up a world and make it real.

A Weekend in the Life

Saturday morning in the hospital. Outside, a hot August day is beginning, cars are already heading out of the city toward the beach, people in bed are stretching, remembering it's Saturday, rolling over to sleep for a few hours more. But in the hospital, the lights are fluorescent, the climate is controlled, and the day is beginning. On the fifth floor, Team 2 is convening for work rounds, a resident, two interns, two medical students.

"It's going to be a beautiful day," one of the interns mutters to the medical students. "I am always, and I mean always, on call when the weather is good."

As the group hurries off down the hall to begin rounds, one medical student says to the other, "Oh God, I don't want to be here this morning."

Internship is the first year after medical school. All internships begin in July, so in August, all the interns have been doctors for a month or so. They are just barely accustomed to writing "M.D." after their names, and they are profoundly aware of their limited experience, their limited knowledge in a profession in which it is impossible to know it all. They depend on the people above them in the hierarchy to save them from the possible results of limited experience and limited knowledge. The resident has already finished internship; he directs the team and oversees the interns. The interns and the residents together constitute the house staff. And the medical students are wetting their feet for the first time, in the hospital to learn about the hospital, to watch the interns and imagine themselves doing that job, as they will be, in a couple of years.

The resident is John McGonigle. He is quite small, thin and wiry, with curly red hair; he almost dances through the hospital, and his ironic nickname among the interns and residents is Godzilla. His style is brusque and rapid-paced; he likes to imagine his team rolling quickly along, making decisions, firing snappy insults at one another, and, if possible, making it to the cafeteria before breakfast is over. He is very fond of cheese Danish. Twenty-nine years old, this month he will put in about 130 hours a week, in a position of tremendous responsibility, and earn something over $24,000 a year.

The intern on call for the day is Phil Maxwell, a blond twenty-seven-year-old hotshot from the Midwest, open-faced, blue-eyed, and profoundly compulsive. Even among the house staff, where people proudly acknowledge themselves as type A's, Phil has the reputation of going a little too far, working a little too hard. The intern who is post-call, who has heen in the hospital all night, is Karen Newton, thirty years old; she has curly brown hair and tired brown eyes. She did research for a couple of years at the end of medical school, got an MD-PhD, and though she is respected by the house staff for the important papers which are now being published with her name on them, she is also known to be a little rusty at clinical work; all that time in the lab. The interns don't work quite as many hours as the resident this month, since they get days off now and then. Say 115 hours a week. They make about $22,000 a year.

That leaves the two medical students. They work

with the interns, so one of them is post-call, and one of them is on call. The post-call student is Matthew Baxter; it is no coincidence that his name is the same as the name of one of the hospital buildings, generally referred to as "Baxterville." Matthew is to be the fourth generation of brilliant physicians in his family, and since they have been associated with this hospital for over a century, he has very little choice about where he will do his residency. Fortunately, he is an extremely reverent young man, and it has apparently never occurred to him to resent his manifest destiny. Like Karen, he has been up most of the night, preparing one of his customary superb workups on the patient he admitted, and also helping with blood drawing, errands, whatever came along. The other medical student, the one who is on call for the night to come, is more than a little like me. Her hair is pinned up in a bun, her earrings are maybe a little inappropriately large for the hospital (they sometimes clink against her stethoscope and make it hard to hear heart sounds), and she looks a little bit tense and a little bit depressed. It was, needless to say, she and not Matthew who complained of not wanting to be here. We can call her Elizabeth, which is, in fact, my middle name. The medical students are following the interns' schedule, about 115 hours a week. They are each paying $14,000 a year for the privilege.

Work rounds: this is the time for the intern who was on call to bring the team up to date on all the patients, both the old ones, who may have gotten worse overnight, and the new ones she has admitted. The team moves along the hall, pausing in front of every door for Karen to give them a few lines on the patient within.

"Mr. Harrison, definitely ruled out for an MI, spiked to a hundred three last night, I cultured him up, nothing on his chest film, might just be the flu." [Mr. Harrison has been determined not to have had a heart attack (myocardial infarction), had a temperature of 103 last night, got specimens of his blood and his urine sent to the lab to be cultured for bacteria, and has no pneumonia or other problems showing up on his chest X ray.]

"Mrs. Kaplan, stable, awaiting placement." [Mrs. Kaplan is ready to leave the hospital but has nowhere to go, Social Service needs to find a place for her in a nursing home.]

"New admission, Mr. Russo is a sixty-six-year-old white COPDer with multiple admits here, who presented yesterday with increased DOE, admitted to juggle his meds around. He's been intubated twice in the past. . . ." [Mr. Russo is a sixty-six-year-old white man with chronic obstructive pulmonary disease who has been in this hospital many times and came in yesterday with increased dyspnea (shortness of breath) on exertion and was admitted so we could adjust his drug regimen. He has needed a breathing tube and a ventilator twice in the past. . . .]

The resident, John McGonigle, makes notes about each new patient on a new file card, updates his file cards on the old patients. He is responsible for all these people; if the intern has made a mistake, this is his first opportunity to catch it. He occasionally raps out a question, as about Mr. Harrison: "Did you look at his sputum?"

"He wasn't really bringing anything up," Karen says, not adding that she was much too busy last night to stand around waiting for someone to cough up some sputum, and then go prepare and stain slides in the lab and hunt for bugs under the microscope.

"I could check that later, if you want," offers Matthew Baxter; sputum examination is frequently a medical student job. Elizabeth feels a very slight and completely unreasonable irritation at his eager-beaver manner.

The team finishes rounds, and does indeed make it down to the cafeteria in time for breakfast; John gets his Danish and everyone else gets coffee and rather uninspiring scrambled eggs. The food is eaten quickly, and conversation is restricted to the events of the previous night on the ward.

Attending rounds: the attending is the senior physician responsible for supervising the team. He comes in every day except Sunday to hear about new admissions, teach the students, advise on complicated cases. The attending is Dr. Harry Black, a soft-spoken man with a rather distressing talent for going off on tangents, but a good and humane doctor.

Matthew Baxter presents his patient, a twenty-seven-year-old black woman who came to the hospital with a vague history of fatigue, weight loss, stomach pains—and in the emergency room, the intern examining her felt an enormously enlarged liver. So now she is in the hospital to be worked up, and Matthew runs down a list of possible diagnoses: hepatitis, other infections, malignancies. Dr. Black, after listening to the details of the case, announces that he would personally put his money on malignancy.

John McGonigle's eyes light up at this turn of phrase. "What kind?" he wants to know. He proposes a bet: is this a primary liver cancer, is it a metastasis from a gut cancer, or from a lung tumor, or from a breast tumor?

Dr. Black, who is perhaps now a little uncomfortable with this talk of betting, turns to the medical students and asks suddenly, "What other cancer commonly metastasizes to the liver, and why is it unlikely in this patient?"

Elizabeth has no idea, though she thinks quickly of a likely guess, but Matthew has been up all night reading about liver disease, and says quickly, "Melanoma, very unusual in blacks."

But John McGonigle is attached to the idea of a bet, and is in addition not unwilling to struggle a little with the attending for control of rounds, so he persists: a bottle of wine to the person who correctly names the malignancy. He himself will go for gut metastasis, and Matthew Baxter, eager to please his resident, immediately claims primary liver cancer, since some people think that is associated with the birth control pill and this patient, Mrs. Ropers, has taken the Pill in the past. Phil Maxwell, looking a little bored, says that in that case he'll go with lung tumor, which leaves Karen and Elizabeth, the two women, with breast, and that makes everyone slightly uncomfortable. Nevertheless, John writes out a list, more than a little tickled.

The team briefly discusses one other new admission, a diabetic man named Mr. Theokratis, visiting from California, sixty years old, who seems to have had a very bad attack of his customary asthma. Karen Newton explains that though both Mr. Theokratis and his wife were a little frightened by the severity of the episode, it is something that has apparently happened many times before, and Mr. Theokratis is looking much better already this morning. "He may be ready to go home tomorrow," she adds.

Attending rounds are over and the real work of the day begins. Because it is Saturday, there are no conferences; also because it is Saturday, most tests are not available except in cases of emergency. For their investigative CAT scans, their barium swallows, their echocardiographies, their pulmonary function tests, the patients will wait for next week. The team will try to keep them stable, get them through the weekend, and where further diagnostic workups are needed, pick those workups up again in a couple of days.

Matthew Baxter goes in to get an arterial blood gas on Mr. Theokratis, to measure the amount of oxygen in his blood. Because getting blood from an artery means a much more painful needle stick than in a regular blood-drawing from a vein, some people inject a little local anesthetic into the skin of the wrist before aiming the needle directly down at the beating pulse. Matthew, however, prefers not to do this, on the perfectly reasonable grounds that it means two needle sticks instead of one, and in addition the local anesthetic can mean a little swelling in the area of the wrist, making it that much harder to hit the artery on the first try. However, Mr. Theokratis is an old veteran of arterial blood gas samples; the first thing he says when he sees the syringe is, "Get some Xylocaine, young man, or you don't come anywhere near me."

Obligingly, Matthew gets the Xylocaine, injects it, and then, sure enough, it takes him two attempts to get the needle into the artery. When he finally hits it, and the red blood begins to spurt into the syringe, powered by the strong arterial pulse, Mr. Theokratis says sourly, "You need a little more practice, sonny." Matthew, who has after all been up almost all night, feels a sudden urge to say, well, next time you want anesthetic you can whistle for it. But instead he smiles, pulls out the needle, and presses a gauze pad over he site of the puncture with one hand, while with the other he removes the needle from the now full syringe, attaches a small rubber cap in its place, and rolls the syringe back and forth between his thumb and forefinger so the blood will mix well with the anticlotting substance in the tube. The syringe full of blood goes into a bag of ice, the pressure is applied to Mr. Theokratis's wrist for the specified five minutes, and then Matthew leaves the room, depositing the sample at the ward secretary's desk. The ward secretary calls for a transporter to come take it down to the lab.

Because it is Saturday, John McGonigle sends his postcall intern home soon after noon. Karen Newton is now free for the rest of the day and for Sunday as well; since she is neither on call nor post-call, she doesn't have to come in. This adds up to one day off every three weeks, and Karen is profoundly grateful to John for letting her out so early, increasing her daylight time out of the hospital by fifty percent. Sure, she thinks, Godzilla may be a bit much at times, but he does take care of his people. And before anything can come up requiring her help, she grabs her stethoscope and leaves. She is going home to a couple of weeks of undone laundry, promising herself a phone call to her boyfriend from medical school, who is in a city a thousand miles away doing a surgical residency— he'll be in the hospital, of course, but even in surgery things can be slow on a Saturday, so she'll page him. And she is also going home to a whole free Sunday, and she knows from past experience that she will never be able to come up with an activity momentous enough, joyous enough, worthy of that day outside the hospital.

John tells Matthew Baxter that he should hurry up and write notes on all his patients and get the hell out of the hospital; he too is off Sunday. Matthew, however, is very anxious that no one should see him as unenthusiastic, or eager to leave, so he says, cheerfully, "That's fine, but I'm having a good time." He is immediately conscious that everyone listening thinks he is talking like a fool, and he blushes, then goes off to see his new patient, Mrs. Ropers. An eager-beaver medical student may impress a senior physician, too far from medical school to remember the tricks of the trade, but the house staff looks on someone who spends extra unnecessary hours in the hospital as mentally defective.

Elizabeth goes down to collect the midday printouts

of lab results on the bloods drawn early that morning. As she rides up in the elevator from the basement labs, she looks over the printout, wondering whether all these numbers will ever be clear and obvious to her. Her fears about her own lack of knowledge, her inability to think sanely and straightforwardly about a set medical problem, are always part of her approach to the hospital. She is stuffed full of facts, memorized and partly remembered, from her medical school courses. She has learned a certain amount in the hospital, idiosyncratically absorbed according to her own interest in certain patients, her level of alertness on morning rounds on some particular mornings, the articulateness of the people doing the teaching.

She runs her finger across the printout, trying to convince herself that the numbers are speaking to her and she is understanding their message. So this patient's liver function tests are slightly up from yesterday, up just above the edge of normal. Does that mean anything? Probably not. Suddenly she notices something in Mr. Theokratis's results, looks again, double-checks against the list of normal lab values on the back of the printout.

When she gets off the elevator at the fifth floor, she finds Phil Maxwell, her intern, and shows him the printout, asking, almost timidly, "Doesn't it look like Mr. Theokratis is having an MI?"

Phil grabs the printout away from her and stares at it. A cardiac enzyme, creatinine phosphokinase (CPK), is sharply elevated in Mr. Theokratis's blood, and this enzyme is usually elevated right after a heart attack.

"I can't believe they didn't check this out last night in the emergency room," Phil says to Elizabeth, as the two of them hurry along the corridor to find John. "This was really careless of Karen; when you're dealing with a diabetic, you have to allow for the possibility of a painless MI, they have them all the time."

They find John, and Phil thrusts the printout at him, his finger indicating the value.

"Oh, shit!" says John McGonigle.

An hour later, Mr. Theokratis is in the intensive care unit, and Team 2 is no longer responsible for his well-being. John and Phil are arguing about what the proper course of treatment and diagnosis would have been the night before, when Mr. Theokratis showed up with his story of an asthma attack like a hundred other asthma attacks. It is not completely possible to tell, of course, whether he was really having an asthma attack, and had a heart attack maybe brought on by the strain of it, or whether his difficulty breathing was actually attributable all along to his painless heart attack. One way or another, no one thought much about a heart attack last night, since the asthma therapy seemed to make him better; his electrocardiogram was very nonspecific, and the cardiac enzyme values didn't come back from the lab until morning.

John McGonigle is annoyed to have a heart attack discovered like this; he feels it looks bad for his team. Phil Maxwell is convinced that it wouldn't have happened if he had been on call. He reassures himself of this several times, waiting for John to chime in, agree that Karen made an obvious mistake, even if he is not quite sure what the mistake was. John, whose opinion of all interns is low (he finished his own internship only a month ago, and it is important to him to set himself apart from those lowly ignorant beginners), offers no such agreement.

Elizabeth goes to see a patient she has been following for quite a while, an elderly gentleman named Mr. Wissel. He came into the hospital almost two months ago for some fairly minor urinary tract surgery. Following his surgery, he developed pneumonia, and after that his wound from the surgery began to look infected. To make matters worse, he picked up a urinary tract infection. The urological surgeons have finally handed him over to the medical team, essentially washing their hands of him. Nothing that has happened to him is particularly surprising; hospital-acquired infections are a very common problem, especially in elderly or debilitated patients. Mr. Wissel has just had a particularly bad run of them. In addition, like many elderly people, he has found the hospital extremely disorienting and confusing, and whether from that alone or from drug side effects as well, he is no longer mentally intact. When he came to the hospital, he was a pleasant, reasonably sharp gentleman who lived alone and did his own shopping and cooking. He still has days on which he is more or less with it, but he also has many days when he seems completely disconnected from everything going on around him, when he becomes abusive, or seems to suffer from delusions. He is now classified as needing "placement." His current major problem is a pneumonia that seems to come back every time he finishes a course of antibiotics aimed at eradicating it. Elizabeth takes a sample of his sputum every day and stains it, looks at it under the microscope to see what she can see. Usually nothing, but it makes her feel as if she is at least trying to do *something* for poor Mr. Wissel, who, when he is not totally out of it, is really a very sweet, if somewhat lecherous, old man. The nurse has a little vial of sputum ready for Elizabeth, and she goes and shuts herself in the little closet of a lab, smears the admittedly rather disgusting stuff on a slide, stains it with the various reagents of the Gram's stain, puts it under the microscope. She makes her usual diagnosis, shmutz, and reports it to John.

Matthew Baxter is furious; he has just called down to find out the results of that arterial blood gas he drew on Mr. Theokratis, now very important to know; the intensive care unit team wants those numbers.

And the blood gas lab insists they never received the sample; transport must have lost it—or maybe they dropped it and broke it and didn't want to report it. The unit team will have to draw another. The little, essentially unavoidable mistakes of dropping, losing, mislabeling, misreading which would be taken for granted in many settings can become highly charged in the hospital. The support people, the techs who draw the blood, the transporters who carry it to the lab, the lab techs who do the tests and report them, are often blamed for major medical screwups, sometimes because of small errors they have made, or genuine carelessness, and sometimes because they are an anonymous and convenient scapegoat. Matthew, for example, feels right now that if the transport people had been more careful with Mr. Theokratis's blood gas, maybe . . . well, maybe things would be going better for Mr. Theokratis, that's all, and the unit team, when he tells them about the lost blood gas, curse the transport person as if he had caused the heart attack in the first place.

Phil Maxwell gets called by the intern in the emergency room, who announces that they have two new admissions sitting there waiting for him, the intern on call for Team 2. Phil disappears down toward his new patients, not to be seen on the ward again for several hours.

"Elizabeth, will you please go start a new IV on Mrs. Pinkerton," says John McGonigle. It is getting on toward evening, and he wants to go home. It is Saturday, after all, and he is on call tomorrow night, and though it is sometimes hard to believe it when he is acting like a ten-year-old, Godzilla McGonigle is married, and presumably he likes to see his wife every now and then. In fact, he wants badly to go home and take off his shoes and eat dinner with his wife, but he can't leave until everything with Team 2 is completely stable. And he has to come in every single day. So here he sees his evening (four hours, say, between coming home and going to sleep) being whittled away, and it makes him irritable. And Mrs. Pinkerton is a lady who everyone knows is not going to get better, and she can't feel anything most of the time, and her husband sits over you when you are trying to start an IV on her, muttering, "Oh, be careful! Oh, don't hurt her, please!" So Elizabeth collects her equipment, the IV needle, a tourniquet, alcohol swabs, tape, and goes into Mrs. Pinkerton's room. Now, Mrs. Pinkerton's is a very sad story. She has had severe and inoperable brain metastases, has gone through radiation therapy with no real improvement. She was taken home by her devoted husband to live out her days, but she developed seizures and he had to bring her back in. Her husband haunts the hospital, spending long days by her bedside, talking to her about all the things they will do together, as soon as she is well, how they will visit their children and grandchildren out in Texas, how they will buy new curtains for the living room. Mrs. Pinkerton is kept heavily sedated, and even when she is awake, it is clear enough that she does not understand what is said to her. Sometimes she can respond to simple questions or commands, but that is about it.

"Hello, Doctor," Mr. Pinkerton says to Elizabeth, as she bustles in. Mr. Pinkerton always manages to convey the hope that maybe this time, maybe this doctor, there will be a new treatment, a new answer, a new chance.

"I need to start her IV," Elizabeth says, wrapping the tourniquet around the old woman's wasted arm. Mr. Pinkerton, as usual, hangs forward, telling Elizabeth, "Now, you will be careful, won't you, Doctor? She always had such sensitive skin."

In fact, there have been so many IVs in Mrs. Pinkerton's veins, and her blood vessels in general are so thin and tortuous, that Elizabeth simply cannot see any likely place to put the new IV. And with Mr. Pinkerton sitting so close, she feels extremely reluctant to just poke blindly. She takes off the tourniquet and goes in search of John, wishing that he were gone for the day and Phil left in charge. Phil may be intense, but he is always willing to teach. She could say to him, will you help me find a vein on Mrs. Pinkerton, and he would come and help. But John McGonigle, when she finds him, merely looks at her in exaggerated disbelief and says, "You're in your third year of medical school, you should be able to start an IV. No excuses."

So Elizabeth wheels around and goes back to Mrs. Pinkerton, mentally telling old Godzilla where he gets off. Godzilla, it is only fair to say, is not the least bit interested in teaching. He looks at medical students as conveniences, work-saving devices for his team, but he has no desire to fulfill the other half of the usual bargain, and pay back any of the time they save in teaching. Anyway, right now Godzilla is in no mood to be patient with anyone who may delay him from going home.

It takes Elizabeth four tries to get the IV going, though she frankly doubts whether any of the house staff could have done it more easily; this woman's veins are simply shot to hell. Mr. Pinkerton looks at Elizabeth reproachfully, but he manages gamely, "Thank you very much, Doctor," as she gathers up her wasted needles and leaves.

Matthew Baxter goes home, after writing a two-page progress note on his new patient, Mrs. Ropers, the woman with the big liver. The progress note is a masterpiece of diplomacy, outlining all the possibilities discussed in attending rounds without committing itself to any as more likely than another, despite Matthew's bet on liver cancer. He has also, of course, written notes on all the other patients he is following, and he is getting a little exhausted.

Even John McGonigle goes home, after one last tense conversation with the intensive care unit team about how he could ever have allowed Mr. Theokratis's MI to get by him like that. "Okay, now," John says to Phil Maxwell, "call me if you have any serious problems, but they damn well better be serious." And he goes home to what is really now only a two-and-a-half-hour evening, knowing he will give himself an extra hour or two to enjoy being out of the hospital, and then be tired tomorrow.

Elizabeth is working up her patient for the evening, a twenty-six-year-old man who speaks only Spanish, who has come into the hospital because for the last three days he has had terrible vomiting and diarrhea; he is seriously dehydrated, and the most important thing to do for him is to get some fluid into him. In the emergency room they started his IV (Elizabeth is just as glad not to be doing another one of those right away), and she has some time to find out his history. Unfortunately, her Spanish is very weak, though it is better than Phil Maxwell's; he speaks no Spanish at all, which is why he assigned her to this particular patient. She manages to find out from him how long all this has been going on, whether there has been blood in his stool *("Hay sangre?")* and whether there has been stomach pain *("Hay dolor?"),* and since she knows Phil will ask about this, she attempts to find out his sexual history. After all, if he is gay, there are various intestinal parasites that can be sexually acquired which ought to be included in her list of possible diagnoses, and Phil, after all, is compulsive.

Unfortunately, Elizabeth is unable to make herself understood when she asks this question (all she can manage is to ask if he has female friends—*amigas*— and he says yes, so she asks if he has male friends— *amigos*—and he again says yes, and looks puzzled). She considers drawing pictures, then decides not to pursue it, since, after all, he could also have acquired these intestinal parasites at his home in Mexico, so the sexual history would not really make any difference. Or so she will tell Phil.

She makes sure that her new patient, Mr. Vargas, is comfortably settled in his room, then hurries down to pick up trays for Phil and herself at the free on-call late-night supper being served down in the cafeteria. Egg salad is, after all, better than nothing.

Phil Maxwell by now has five admissions to work up. He examines each patient as thoroughly as possible, carefully runs his mind down a list of the things to be thought of, the things to be done, the diagnoses to be ruled out, the diagnoses to be considered. His write-ups on his patients are marvels of logical organization and clearheaded ratiocination; unfortunately, his handwriting is almost unreadable. He is feeling very pressured by what happened today with Mr. Theokratis. He would like to believe that he could never let a thing like that get by him, that Karen was truly careless last night—but he knows that in fact he could easily let a great many things get by him. Every night on call he sees things he has never seen before; he has, after all, been a doctor for only a month and a half. There are always things to be thought of that he will not think of, there are possibilities too bizarre to worry about that turn out to be facts, and strong probabilities that fail to pan out. He does not actually say to himself, what if I kill someone, but that thought is always in the background of his mind.

In fact, he often finds himself inventing scenarios,

wrong decisions he could make that would leave someone dead or dying. Most of these scenarios involve
being too slow to call for help when he needs it; Phil
the intern is not alone in the hospital at night. A
senior resident, an anesthesiologist, a surgeon, and
various other people are all available if he asks for
them. But if he is too slow to recognize a problem, if
he tries to treat something himself when it is in fact
beyond him—he can make up hundreds of stories with
himself as villain.

He, like many of the other house staff, believes that
the training he is going through is necessay and irre-
placeable. You cannot learn to be a doctor if you are
not left alone to care for patients. But like many of the
other interns, he sometimes finds himself wondering,
especially in the very early hours of the morning,
when he has not slept and will not sleep, whether it is
actually necessary to be left alone so very tired and so
very stressed. This question was actually raised one
morning on attending rounds, when Dr. Black was
asking the interns how they thought they were doing,
whether they were surviving. Dr. Black took the opportunity to reflect at some length on his own training,
which was, as all former initiations always are, much
more rigorous than what kids have to do today. "It
was every other night for three solid years," Dr. Black
told Team 2. "We worked harder than you can imagine. We were like soldiers in the trenches. It was the
best training anyone could ever have."

Phil Maxwell thinks about this, a little sourly, when
the emergency room calls him yet again. He is not at
all pleased to hear about his newest admission. The
Burton family is down in the emergency room; their
twenty-year-old daughter, Eleanor, is dying of bone
cancer, and they have brought her into the hospital
because she is suddenly worse. As on so many other
hospital admissions, they fear, and maybe also hope a

little, that this will be the last one. Eleanor Burton has five volumes of old hospital charts that Phil will have to look at (a less compulsive intern might just glance at the most recent volume), and her family is very used to the hospital; they will not tolerate anything they see as suboptimal care. And in addition, here is this woman, younger than himself, and she is dying of a terrible, horrible disease, one that is on Phil's own personal list of the four or five worst, the shoot-me-if-I-get-like-that diseases, a list maintained by almost all medical personnel.

But Phil is a nice guy, and he extends himself to be kind and comforting to this family, which is essentially beyond comfort, and after he leaves them, he finds he is ravenous. The tray that Elizabeth brought for him is sitting rather disconsolately by the nurses' station, and he eats his egg-salad sandwich in two bites. Then the emergency room calls to tell him about yet another admission.

As he is heading out, he passes Elizabeth, who is writing up her note on Mr. Vargas. He stops, thanks her for the supper, and asks her if she would please give Mrs. Pinkerton a dose of Dilantin, an antiseizure medication. The drug is to be given intravenously, through Mrs. Pinkerton's line, and the nurses are not allowed to give IV drugs, and it is time for the dose, and Phil cannot stay to give it. He reminds Elizabeth that Dilantin has to be given very slowly, taking the patient's blood pressure at intervals while it is being given, since it can cause a sudden drop in pressure.

Mrs. Pinkerton is not actually one of the patients Elizabeth has been following, though of course she knows about her, and she knows her husband; everyone on the ward knows Mr. Pinkerton, with his gifts of cake and flowers, his embarrassing gratitude when after all they cannot make his wife better. Elizabeth has never given any Dilantin to anyone before, but the nurse helps her draw up the correct dose and warns her once again about giving it slowly and checking the blood pressure. Elizabeth does as she is told, but, to her horror, when she checks the pressure after the third tiny increment of drug, the pressure is way down. She grabs the phone by the bed and pages Phil Maxwell, tells him what is happening, and asks him to come right away.

"Okay, calm down," Phil says. "She's DNR anyway, isn't she?"

Mr. Pinkerton had heen persuaded, though he was quite reluctant to agree, that it would be madness to subject his wife to cardiopulmonary resuscitation, to a mechanical ventilator, to electric shocks to the heart. Still, Elizaheth is not prepared to see her injection of Dilantin as a mercy killing.

"Come up here," she says to Phil with a certain amount of fury in her voice. She can just imagine herself facing Mr. Pinkerton tomorrow, after injecting the Dilantin too fast and killing his wife.

So Phil comes up, Mrs. Pinkerton gets fluid and medications, her blood pressure comes back up, and she will be as alive tomorrow as she was today. Elizabeth, who is trembling from having almost killed someone, goes back to finish writing her note on Mr. Vargas, telling herself over and over that she had injected the Dilantin just as slowly as she was supposed to, there had been no way to prevent the drop in blood pressure. And there is no way to know, of course, whether she in fact pushed the drug a little too fast, whether the dose she drew up with the nurse was wrong, or whether it is just that this very weak, very sick lady has many reasons for a drop in blood pressure. It is also true that the legal status of medical students in the hospital is very unclear. Are they actually allowed to give IV drugs? Who is liable for their errors? Medical students sometimes end up doing things they aren't sure they're supposed to do simply because they are needed, the intern is frantically busy, the patient is sick . . .

The night goes on. Mr. Vargas, who is fundamentally healthy, begins feeling much better after only a few hours of intravenous fluids. Mr. Wissel wakes up and becomes first lucid, and then somewhat deranged, shouting obscenities at the nurses. They have a standing order for tranquilizers on him, since this has happened before, and they medicate him back into his dreams. Eleanor Burton is fighting her last battle, and her parents, veterans of many stays in this hospital, are sitting in her room, though visiting hours are of course long over; the nurses know them well, and everyone feels they are entitled to be there. Up in the intensive care unit, Mr. Theokratis suffers yet another painless heart attack; this time, because he is so thoroughly monitored, everyone knows exactly what is going on, but they feel a little less superior to John McGonigle and his team, since even with all their elaborate monitoring equipment, they were unable to prevent this. Mrs. Pinkerton stares up at the ceiling, seeing nothing. And Mrs. Ropers, the woman with the liver, gets a fever.

It is three o'clock in the morning. Elizabeth has just climbed into the top bunk in the on-call room, after spending an hour reading about all the various causes of gastroenteritis, with blood in the stool and without, with vomiting and without, and so on. She is beginning to have unpleasant dreams about stomach cramps when Phil comes in and wakes her, apologizing, tells her that Mrs. Ropers has spiked a temp and he, Phil, has three IVs to start on other patients. So Elizabeth gets up and goes to draw blood cultures on Mrs. Ropers to check for infections in the blood. Elizabeth and Phil by now are both wearing green cotton surgical scrubs, the pajamas of the hospital. Elizabeth draws the blood reasonably efficiently, scrubbing off the skin where she means to draw it with several washes of disinfectant so the cultures will not be contaminated with skin bacteria, changing her needle before she shoots the blood into the culture bottles so the culture will not be contaminated if there are a few skin bugs on the needle. Then Mrs. Ropers gets some Tylenol, and goes off to sleep, and eventually Elizabeth climbs back up into the top bunk and does the same.

Phil Maxwell does not go to sleep. He has notes to write on his total of six admissions, and he is quite concerned about a couple of seriously ill patients—Mr. Russo, for example, the COPDer who was admitted the night before. His respiratory status is deteriorating, and Phil has to decide when and if it gets bad enough for him to require intubation—always a dangerous thing in a patient like this one, who may never come off the vent. Phil goes and checks on him every so often, considers changes he might make in his medications. The senior resident who is on call for the whole hospital to help with tricky patients comes by, looks Mr. Russo over with Phil, agrees with everything Phil is doing, and leaves, telling him he's managing this perfectly, he doesn't need any help. This is meant to bolster Phil's confidence, of course, to take him one step closer to independence as a doctor, and in fact Phil is pleased to hear it, though still frightened to be left in charge.

And then there is Mrs. Ropers; tired as he is, Phil wants to give some thought to her liver, not the kind of cursory nonsense that went on in rounds. Phil feels that Dr. Black is allowing John McGonigle to get away with altogether too much at attending rounds; Godzilla needs to be kept in hand. This silliness about betting, for example—this would have been an excellent teaching case if Godzilla hadn't sidetracked everyone with his nonsense. It's a fascinating diagnostic question, especially in this young woman who doesn't really fit the profile for any of the malignancies. If Phil had time, he would like to read through her chart carefully, do a complete physical exam himself. But he doesn't have time, of course. And now she has a fever. He thinks about possible causes for fever, all the obvious infections, the fever mysteriously associated with malignancy—tumor fever. Then he goes back to his notes. He is still sitting at the nurses' station, writing, when John McGonigle arrives the next morning for work rounds.

On Sunday, the attending does not come in. Work rounds are quickly over, and Phil gets to go home almost immediately. John also sends Elizabeth home early; by tradition, those who are on call Saturday night get some of Sunday off. John McGonigle will manage the ward alone for that day and night.

The day is comparatively quiet, a few new admissions, none of them terribly sick. Mrs. Ropers continues to run a temperature whenever she doesn't get her Tylenol, and John is unable to find a source of infection, so he doesn't have anything to treat. Mr. Russo does not have to be intubated after all, which John views as a personal triumph; he doesn't want to lose any more patients to the intensive care unit. When he runs into the unit team, he teases them without mercy for letting Mr. Theokratis have another MI.

Pretty weak, guys," he says, over and over; this is his ultimate insult.

Mrs. Pinkerton stays at her usual level, Mr. Vargas is quickly getting better. There may never be a clear answer to what caused Mr. Vargas's diarrhea; something may grow on stool culture, or it may not. In any case, John speaks only enough Spanish to conduct a very basic physical exam (*"Respire profundo!"*—Breathe deeply), so he doesn't spend any time talking to Mr. Vargas. Or to Mrs. Pinkerton, who of course doesn't talk, or to Mr. Pinkerton, who is always trying to engage him in deeply respectful conversation. Or with Eleanor Burton, a clear and obvious goner.

And now Mr. Wissel, another gorked-out old gomer. The nurses have come to tell John that Mr. Wissel is complaining again, pains in his head, pains in his stomach, his children never come to visit him. They want to know if John would give him a stronger tranquilizer, which John does. Mr. Wissel settles down uneasily. John also begins to feel uneasy about this a little while later; he recalls hearing it mentioned on rounds that Mr. Wissel has been complaining of stomach pains on and off for a couple of days. Maybe just as well to have a better look at him.

Unfortunately, between Mr. Wissel's mental state and the heavy load of tranquilizers and sedatives, it's hard for John to be sure about the abdominal exam— does this hurt? does this hurt? how about if I press here? He spends a long time going over Mr. Wissel's abdomen, and finally satisfies himself that it does in fact feel suspicious. So John calls for an emergency X ray, which also looks suspicious. He is angry at himself for medicating the patient without properly examining him, and he elects to blame this on the nurses, who he feels did not keep him properly informed. He gives Mr. Wissel's nurse a short and unpleasant lecture, the gist of which is, you may have killed this patient. The nurse, who has been a nurse for almost fifteen times as long as John has been a doctor, is not unduly upset by this; John is a notorious jerk when it comes to dealing with nurses. *"You're* supposed to be the doctor," she tells him. "Too bad if it's too much for you."

John's mood has not improved as he calls in the surgeons, announces to them, this is one of the guys you screwed up but good, and now he has intestinal obstruction, so you damn well better cure it.

The surgeons, though they agree that it looks like obstruction, are very reluctant to operate, pointing out that Mr. Wissel is very debilitated and that his mental function is hardly what you would call intact.

Suddenly John McGonigle is in a fury. "Now, listen to me," he almost shouts at the surgeons. "This guy *walked* into this hospital. Do you hear me, he walked in, he was okay except for some little plumbing problem, and then the asshole surgeons got hold of him and since then it's been urinary tract infection and wound infection and pneumonia and bedsores and all the rest, and you can goddam well take him to surgery and try to help him out." John rather enjoys a good fit of anger; he has never been particularly interested in Mr. Wissel before, but he is happy to be telling the surgeons where to get off.

"Okay, Godzilla, just relax," the surgeons tell him. Ultimately, they agree to take Mr. Wissel to the operating room. As they leave the ward, one of the surgical interns, a woman, says to the senior surgical resident, "Well, old Godzilla was certainly on the rag today." This does not improve John's temper.

John is impatient with paperwork, and when he sends down a tube of Mr. Wissel's blood to the blood bank so that they can match it with some blood to transfuse during surgery, he neglects to stamp up all the proper forms and labels that have to go to the blood bank. A surgeon calls, an hour later, to tell John rather gleefully that the blood bank has thrown away the improperly labeled tube and John will have to draw more blood. The blood bank is extremely picky about this, since giving someone blood that was meant for another patient could easily be fatal; unless all the stamps and identification numbers are there, no blood is matched. Cursing, John draws more blood, then asks a nurse to stamp and label the tube. The nurses do not generally like John, who is none too polite with them, but they are on his side in the matter of Mr. Wissel, whom they rather like, so no one minds helping out with the blood.

After that, it's a quiet night, no new admissions after eleven o'clock; John writes up short notes (no one is going to criticize *him,* after all) and gets a reasonable amount of sleep.

On Monday morning, just as work rounds are beginning, Eleanor Burton dies. Phil Maxwell, the intern who admitted her, finds himself awkwardly trying to comfort her parents, who are torn between relief that her miseries are over, and the grief they are finally letting out about her entire illness.

"Listen," says John McGonigle, "we've gotta start rounds. Call up their usual doc, Shlepperman, and get him over here. He's the one they need to see."

Phil Maxwell, who is, after all, from the Midwest, begins paging through the hospital phone book, looking for Shlepperman. Elizabeth waits until John is out of hearing, and then suggests, "I think the name is actually Klepperman." Phil finds the name, pages Dr. Klepperman, grateful that he doesn't have to go back in to the Burtons himself.

The week has begun, and morning rounds are brisk and efficient. Matthew Baxter is eager to get to work on establishing the diagnosis on Mrs. Ropers. Karen Newton, knowing she is on call today, has the wound-up, tensed look of someone who is prepared not to relax for thirty-six hours. John McGonigle leads them all rapidly through the corridors, demonstrating his idea of how things ought to be done: see how smoothly things go when *I'm* on call? Phil Maxwell and Elizabeth are happy in the position of people with a good night's sleep behind them and the prospect of another tonight; true only one day out of every three.

Mr. Wissel is in the recovery room, after his surgery. His condition is tenuous. Mrs. Pinkerton is staring at the ceiling. Her condition is stable. Mr. Vargas is almost completely better, even feeling a little hungry today. Mr. Russo is also much better, moving steadily toward leaving the hospital; he will not stay out for long, of course, but he looks forward to going home. Mr. Theokratis, up in the unit, is doing amazingly well; he still refuses to believe he had even one heart attack, and he laughs at the doctors when they try to tell him that he will have to take special care of his heart from now on. Eleanor Burton is dead; her medical history is resolved, and her story is ended. And Mrs. Ropers is lying in bed, spiking her mysterious temperatures, with her mysterious big liver. Her medical history is only beginning.

Match Day

Perhaps this March 19 didn't mean anything special to you. Maybe you had a child applying to college and were focused on April 15. Or maybe you had nothing momentous pending this spring. But for most of us in our fourth year of medical school, March 19 was Match Day, and nothing has been the same since.

Every June new doctors graduate from medical schools across America, and somehow they have to be sorted into the hospitals in which they will continue their training, as interns in surgery, internal medicine, pediatrics, whatever. Every medical student needs a place (the MD alone does not qualify you to practice medicine), and every teaching hospital needs a full set of interns to take care of patients and generally to keep the place running. And so we have the Match, a national computerized sorting system. Earlier in the year we chose our specialties, applied to various programs, and traveled around the country for interviews, attempting to look like people dying for the opportunity to work more than a hundred hours a week. We came up with polite answers to direct questions ("Do you really want to come here?") and less direct questions ("What are you looking for in your medical education?"), we wore suits and toured one hospital after another, and we questioned interns in all the programs ("What time do you get to leave the day after you're on call?").

And then finally we submitted our rank lists, rating programs in the order in which we desired them, and all the programs submitted ranked lists of applicants, and a computer did the work. So for a couple of months before March 19, whenever I met a friend from medical school, we talked about who had ranked what program first, who had received what kind of encouragement from where, and so on. It's forbidden for the hospitals to tell applicants where they stand, but in fact a great deal of vague unofficial notification goes on.

The day before Match Day I woke up from an anxiety dream; I'd been searching through empty rooms at school to find some very important event that was taking place without me, in a room I couldn't locate. I went to the class I was taking, told a few people about my dream, heard about their dreams. Talked to somebody who had ranked programs in both medicine and surgery and so was waiting to find out not only where he would be but also what he would be. Talked to someone else who had ranked a certain program first but no longer wanted to go there, figured she wouldn't get in if a certain other student in our class did. Calculated our own and everyone else's odds.

Match Day. It is traditional for those who are matching to bring along their spouses and what the medical school chooses to call their semispouses (also known as "significant others"). People bring their children. Everyone's fate is being decided, so everyone comes to see.

The envelopes are made available at noon in Boston; in Chicago they're available at 11:00 A.M. to compensate for the time difference, and so on across the country: all students receive the news at the same moment. At noon, we lined up and got our envelopes, tore them open on the spot or took them out into the hall, hid in the bathroom or in deserted upstairs classrooms, opened them and found out where we'd be for the next three to five years, where we'd train, where we'd live. Much hugging and congratulating, and a photographer who kept trying to take pictures of the people with children (my own child was howling because he'd wanted to open my envelope and I'd been in too much of a hurry to wait while he worked it open).

And after Match Day, things feel different. The transition, which has been for the past four years almost impossible to imagine, has suddenly become real. We're all going to be doctors. When you have the name of the hospital, you can picture yourself working there. Not as a medical student, as a doctor.

At the beginning of medical school I had a tendency to scribble down every stray piece of clinical information that happened to emerge in a lecture. Most of what we heard was "basic science," and pretty far removed from the hospital, but if some lecturer chanced to bring up a disease, a treatment, a risk factor, I wanted to make sure I had it on paper. My brother once said to me, not joking, that if he went to medical school, he'd be afraid to fall asleep in a lecture, afraid he'd miss something vital, which would one day lead to his killing someone. Of course I've become a bit more blase over the past four years (I regularly and deliberately fall asleep in lectures and seminars in the hospital, fighting for my seat in the valued last row, where you can lean your head back against the wall, where the lecturer can't see you so clearly). I've come to understand that left to my own devices and my own knowledge, I would kill many people, no matter how hard I studied; a residency program is designed to keep me from overreaching my experience while at the same time nudging that experience gently along into realms of greater responsibility.

But the point is that even as I became more comfortable sleeping in lectures, I still regarded it as my responsibility to learn something about any given medical topic, and so, I think, did most of my classmates. I'm going to be a doctor and that's a disease—of course I have to know what it is. Well, no more. Ever since Match Day, I feel completely allied to my chosen field—pediatrics. With a smirk, I say to friends going into adult medicine, *"Klebsiella* pneumonia in the debilitated alcoholic—that's your territory, not mine."

"I'm not even going to that lecture," says a classmate. "Malaria is not what I'd call a *surgical* disease."

Although many of us have known for quite a while what we were going into, we seem now to have pledged exclusive allegiance in a new and forceful way. Recently I was in a discussion section where we were evaluating the case of a fifty-five-year-old woman with mysterious fevers and gastrointestinal symptoms. "Run her bowel," suggested a future radiologist, meaning a series of X rays. "Call in the surgeons," suggested someone who had matched in surgery. I looked across the table at another future pediatrician, and we shrugged. "Ear infection, put her on Amoxicillin," I whispered, suggesting a common diagnosis for a two-year-old with fever.

I don't know all that much more than I knew a few months ago; certainly, I haven't made some quantum jump in knowledge that brings me closer to competence as a pediatrician. But I have begun to identify myself completely with the group I'll be joining in July. In part, I suppose this is jubilation—I'm really going to graduate, I really matched, I'm really going to be a doctor. In part, it's probably also fear; in the midst of my terror at having to get out there and be a doctor, it's reassuring to remind myself that there are certain things I don't have to do, certain things I don't have to know. I can worry about whether I'll be competent in pediatrics, and not worry about how much

surgery I do or don't know. I can limit my worrying to
the specific kinds of emergencies I may have to deal
with in a couple of months, and allow myself to write
off areas that would be very important in other fields
of medicine—coronary artery disease, say, or lung cancer. Instead, I have to worry about whether I know
enough about congenital heart disease or leukemia,
the things that affect children—it's still overwhelming,
I'll never know enough, but at least it's limited.

But it isn't just the feeling that *I'm* going to be a
doctor that has affected me since Match Day; it's the
awareness that we're *all* going to be doctors. That
young man who once gave me such complete misinfor-
mation about how the nervous system worked (I believed it, so did he; nonetheless we both did brilliantly
on the test) is going to be in a prestigious medical
residency. The stable people and the unstable ones,
the private people and the people whose every affair is
a medical school event, the people who seem to know
what they're doing and the people who always looked
dazed or blank—they've all been sorted into residencies, they'll all be doctors.

I don't mean to suggest that they're unfit. It's just
that I know who they are. I know how little (or how
much) they know, because we've all had substantially
the same education. I know how big some of our gaps
can be. "I always meant to learn the kidney before I
graduated from medical school," one of my classmates
told me, worriedly. "But the thing is, I really want to
take May off to travel." I knew what he meant. I feel
that way about the liver: a big black box. Ask me
about the liver, I'll give you my grandmother's recipe
(sorry, medical student joke). It's not that any of us
wants to stay in medical school any longer. Quite aside
from the cost, and the human urge to crawl a little way
up the totem pole (though goodness knows interns are
only a couple of millimeters above the mud), we've

had enough of being in school. You can't learn to be a doctor in school; you need an apprenticeship. You need to have responsibility for patients. And in fact, we're all itching to get out there and be doctors. But it still feels amazing to realize that we are all *going* to be doctors, that if you get sick in July, we'll be seeing you.

Conclusion—Baby Doctor

I am going to be a pediatrician. This is a decision that I started to make even before I had done any pediatrics. During my first three months in the hospital, my general medicine clerkship, I became aware that something was wrong. I was not finding clinical medicine as interesting or as rewarding as I had hoped to. It was more interesting to take care of patients than it had been to memorize diseases for a test, but it wasn't fascinating and all-absorbing—as I had sort of hoped it would be. This, after all, was the big apple, the goal of all those courses, the hospital ward. Why wasn't I more involved, more excited about what I was doing? Some of the answer had to do with my circumstances, the particular hospital I had been assigned to, some of the people with whom I had to work closely, some of those who were supposedly teaching me. But I also began to wonder whether I might prefer working with pediatric patients.

And sure enough, when I got to pediatrics I loved it. I was even reasonably happy most of the time—which is not bad for someone who is in the hospital all day every day and all night every fourth night. I felt profoundly involved with my team, with my patients.

The kind of adult medicine I was exposed to in a famous teaching hospital does not of course represent all adult medicine. But when I did adult medicine, we seemed to spend a great deal of our time fighting to save people who have very very limited prospects. A nursing home would send in an elderly patient who had not walked or talked in two years, who had developed a temperature. A person with a rare and fascinating case of something or other would be referred in for more tests—there would be nothing in particular we could do to help, but everyone would repeat, like a mantra, "Great teaching case." In addition, many of the patients had problems that required other kinds of interventions besides medical treatment—people with chronic lung disease who couldn't stop smoking, for example. As doctors, or medical students, we had to leave these things alone; they were outside our domain, and besides, who had time to talk about smoking or diet or exercise or stress? There are, of course, doctors who address all these subjects, but from my point of view it was just another frustration.

But this may all be rationalizing. It's true that in pediatrics you are almost always fighting a battle for a whole lifetime. It's true that you deal much less in what are unfairly stigmatized as "self-induced" problems—the effects of smoking, drinking. (I don't mean to belittle the suffering these substances cause, or imply that sufferers are not entitled to good medical care. I just didn't really get much satisfaction myself from dealing with these problems.) It's also true that in pediatrics you never get to ignore what we rather pompously call the psychosocial aspect of your patients; you always have to deal with the parents, who provide you with the kind of context which is often missing in adult medicine. But maybe what I really discovered about myself was that I like children, as a group, much better than I like adults. And I also tend to like pediatricians more than I like other doctors. I like them because they are not able to be stiff—the adult doctor can stride grandly into the patient's room and announce, we have decided to do this and that, and command respect from many patients. The pediatrician who says, apologetically, to a small patient that such and such a procedure is necessary and will only hurt a tiny bit, is frequently bitten or kicked.

Of course, since I had my own child during medical school, and he has grown to the ripe and stubborn age of two and a half while I was a student, I have had a certain amount of contact with pediatrics from the parent's side of the examining table. When I was applying for residency, I tried to pretend that having had a baby naturally gifted me with tremendous expertise, gave me an advantage over other applicants. This, naturally, was nonsense. Of course, there are a few things I know that come in useful in the hospital. I can change diapers in my sleep, for example. And I know all the developmental milestones, when a child can be expected to smile, walk, talk—except I know them only up as far as Benjamin's age. In other words, I could evaluate any child two and a half or under to see if everything was going on schedule, but I would be lost with three-year-olds (can they build tall towers with blocks? catch baseballs? operate heavy machinery? child-raising is full of surprises). By the end of residency, a three-year process, I expect to be fully competent with any child up to five and a half.

No, the real advantage of having had a child is that I know a great deal more about parents than I otherwise would have. I have brought my own child to the emergency room where I will begin working in a few months, and I will not forget what it felt like to sit in the waiting room, holding a feverish and alarmingly quiet little boy on my lap, wishing that all the other patients would get out of the way so my child could be seen. I have also in my time called the pediatrician because my tiny baby had a funny-looking poop. One night a year or so ago my son had an ear infection, and his temperature went up over 104, and I began to worry that his brain was melting. Now, I happen to know for a fact that brains do not melt; I even had in my notes a lecture I had attended on the syndrome of so-called fever phobia—all the myths parents believe about the ill effects of fever, all the damage they can cause their children by overdosing them with antifever drugs. I read over those notes, then I called the pediatrician and told him that I was worried that my baby's brain might be melting. The doctor on call that night was actually someone who knew me; he had taught me during my pediatrics rotation. And he said to me, gently, come on now, Perri, is this kind of fever really unusual in severe otitis media? And of course I blubbered into the phone, don't ask me any questions, dammit, just tell me my baby is going to be okay, his brain isn't cooking. And does he need a spinal tap? Does he need to be admited to the hospital? And all of this, I suppose, is valuable experience for a pediatrician to have had. Last summer, when I was doing my advanced pediatrics rotation, I admitted a young boy with what we were pretty sure was viral meningitis. We were putting him on antibiotics in case it was bacterial, a much more severe disease, but we weren't really worried. And after I had explained all this to his mother, she suddenly clutched my arm and began to cry. "You can tell me the truth," she sobbed. "He's going to die, he's never going to come out of the hospital alive, is he? My baby's going to die!" It was worth my remembering, right then, despite my impatience that she hadn't heard a word of my brilliant and sensitive explanation, that I am fully capable of the same kind of uncontrollable fears.

Like most medical students, and I suspect like many doctors, I tend to deal with my own illness by denying it. Sometimes I indulge myself, especially if I think I can claim a day off, but basically I don't go to doctors and I don't take medicines—or at least not until I absolutely have to. And as an intern, of course, you aren't allowed to be sick. But for my kid, I am a demanding, frightened, overanxious consumer of medical care. For myself, I accept the various unhealthy constraints of residency—no fresh food, no regular hours, no time for exercise, no stress reduction, no doing any of the things we tell patients to do. But for my kid, I want what everyone wants, healthy circumstances and a life tailored to his needs. So having a child has enlarged my perspective on medicine, and on my chosen branch of medicine in particular, in a number of ways. My son has been and will, I expect, continue to he a steady reminder to me of what my patients represent. They are not their diseases, they are—well, I know what they are. I have one of my own.

And my own reactions to my child have been and will, I expect, continue to be reminders to me of what parents feel when their children are sick, of the hopes, expectations, and fears with which they bring a child to the doctor.

So I am going to be a pediatrician. Two years of preclinical courses, two years of hospital work, and now medical school is ending. I have a great many doubts about the education I have undergone, and most of those doubts are included in these various essays. I do not think my medical education has been extraordinarily well designed, and I think that some of the most effectively conveyed lessons have been the unadvertised teachings about behavior, ethics, style, and power.

As I wrote in the introduction, the process of writing about medical school has changed the last four years for me. I think that in many ways it has helped me through; many of the frustrations and furies of medical school have heen essentially small and petty (it's amazing how petty you can be when you're really tired and you really want to go home), and trying to put my grievances in writing has sometimes helped me sort that out. In the end, I suppose I understand what has happened to me much better for having written about it; there are people who can keep track of themselves without writing anything down, but I am not like that.

I feel obliged to sum it up: am I glad I did it, would I do it again, would I do it differently? I can't answer for myself of four years ago, but I suppose I'm glad, I'd probably do it again. And of course I'd do it differently; I'd do it *right,* whatever that means. I wouldn't let myself be so intimidated, right? I'd defend my dignity, I wouldn't truckle to my superiors, right? I'd really learn everything thoroughly and properly, come out completely *prepared* for internship, right? Well, maybe not.

And so, what I am left with is an appreciation that the last four years have certainly accomplished something. Maybe not all they were intended to accomplish, and maybe also some things they were not meant to do, but one way or another, they have served as an initiation. An initiation of blood (not mine) and pain (mine was the least of it), weariness and confusion, of books and cadavers, needles and plastic tubing, patients and doctors. And I, having been initiated, am left saying, well, here I am—a different person. And, as of this writing, almost but not quite a doctor.

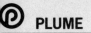 **PLUME**  **MERIDIAN** **DUTTON**

CRITICAL THINKING

☐ **BEYOND CRISIS** *Confronting Health Care in the United States.* **Edited by Nancy F. McKenzie. Foreword by Barbara Ehrenreich.** This timely work provides an unflinching and comprehensive survey of the current state of American health care delivery. There are full examinations of the array of proposals for reform now on the table, including an in-depth look at the Clinton administration's proposed reforms, explorations of the single-payer alternative, as well as sections devoted to community activism and innovations in health care delivery. (011086—$19.95)

☐ **AS REAL AS IT GETS** *The Life of a Hospital at the Center of the AIDS Epidemic.* **by Carol Pogash. Foreword by Randy Shilts.** "An exciting cram course about an invidious disease and about politics and human behavior. The human dimensions of the AIDS epidemic, 'the most important medical story of the century,' grip the reader who comes to know the hospital's doctors, nurses, and patients in this remarkable book."—*Library Journal* (271274—$9.95)

☐ **THE AMERICAN WAY OF BIRTH by Jessica Mitford.** A provocative and entertaining analysis of how and in what circumstances Americans give birth. "An irreverent but honest look at childbirth from the Middle Ages to current times...leaves nothing sacred."—*Boston Sunday Globe* (270685—$12.00)

☐ **ELEMENTAL MIND** *Human Consciousness and the New Physics.* **by Nick Herbert.** Elegantly written and startlingly original, this book offers a new approach to the riddle of consciousness that has challenged philosophers and scientists for centuries. Its implications are nothing short of revolutionary. (935061—$22.00)

Prices slightly higher in Canada.

Buy them at your local bookstore or use this convenient coupon for ordering.

PENGUIN USA
P.O. Box 999, Dept. #17109
Bergenfield, New Jersey 07621

Please send me the books I have checked above.
I am enclosing $_____ (please add $2.00 to cover postage and handling).
Send check or money order (no cash or C.O.D.'s) or charge by Mastercard or VISA (with a $15.00 minimum). Prices and numbers are subject to change without notice.

Card # _____ Exp. Date _____
Signature _____
Name _____
Address _____
City _____ State _____ Zip Code _____

For faster service when ordering by credit card call **1-800-253-6476**

Allow a minimum of 4-6 weeks for delivery. This offer is subject to change without notice

There's an epidemic with 27 million victims. And no visible symptoms.

It's an epidemic of people who can't read.

Believe it *or* not, 27 million Americans are functionally illiterate, about one adult in five.

The solution to this problem is you... when you join the fight against illiteracy. So call the Coalition for Literacy at toll-free **1-800-228-8813** and volunteer.

Volunteer Against Illiteracy. The only degree you need is a degree of caring.